ACTION RESEARCH IN NURSING AND HEALTHCARE

ACTION RESEARCH IN NURSING AND HEALTHCARE

Graham R Williamson
Loretta Bellman
Jonathan Webster

SAGE

Los Angeles | London | New Delhi
Singapore | Washington DC

First published 2012

SAGE Publications Ltd
1 Oliver's Yard
55 City Road
London EC1Y 1SP

SAGE Publications Inc.
2455 Teller Road
Thousand Oaks, California 91320

SAGE Publications India Pvt Ltd
B 1/I 1 Mohan Cooperative Industrial Area
Mathura Road
New Delhi 110 044

SAGE Publications Asia-Pacific Pte Ltd
33 Pekin Street #02-01
Far East Square
Singapore 048763

Library of Congress Control Number: 2011926503

British Library Cataloguing in Publication data

A catalogue record for this book is available from the British Library

ISBN 978-1-84920-001-1
ISBN 978-1-84920-002-8 (pbk)

Typeset by C&M Digitals (P) Ltd, Chennai, India
Printed and bound by CPI group (UK) Ltd, Croydon, CRO 4YY
Printed on paper from sustainable resources

MIX
Paper from responsible sources
FSC® C013604
FSC www.fsc.org

CONTENTS

ABOUT THE AUTHORS

Graham R Williamson is a lecturer in the School of Nursing and Midwifery at Plymouth University. His clinical background is in acute medical nursing and his PhD was an action research study. He is currently co-supervising an action research PhD and has published and presented at conferences on action research issues.

Loretta Bellman has held strategic and operational posts in NHS, university, and independent research organisations. Her main research interests, publications and national and international conference presentations have encompassed applied and practice based research approaches including action research, knowledge transfer and evaluation research. Her doctorate, awarded in 1999, focused on nurse-led change and development in clinical practice using critical action research.

Jonathan Webster qualified as a Registered General Nurse in 1990 and has worked in both secondary and primary care in the UK and Australia. His area of clinical practice is older people's nursing and he has held two Consultant Nurse for Older People posts along with an Assistant Director role for Clinical Quality.

His PhD research focused upon evaluating a programme of emancipatory practice development using action research. Jonathan has written for publication in a variety of professional journals along with presenting at both national and international conferences. His professional, research and scholarship interests lie in developing person-centred ways of working that enable practitioners, teams and organisations to work in partnership with service users and their supporters through practice development and action research.

INTRODUCTION

This book is written for practitioners and academics considering or involved in action research in clinical practice settings. Action research (AR) enables the integration of education, research and clinical practice to advance patient care. In practice disciplines the need for this approach is self-evident, developing personal and professional knowledge and skills while systematically implementing clinical change for patient benefit and involving other practitioners as equal participants. AR is relevant and useful for busy clinicians (including all members of the multidisciplinary health care team who have a direct clinical interface with patients) in affecting change. Managers may find this approach useful for developing services, particularly when there is a focus on quality, improvement, innovation, performance and productivity.

Throughout the book the text has been informed predominantly by the growing action research literature from nursing and healthcare as well as other disciplines, in particular education and management. As this book is focused on the use of action research in clinical settings, we have chosen to refer to this as clinical action research. However, we are in no way trying to create a new action modality within the family of action research (to rank with appreciative inquiry, action science, action inquiry, cooperative inquiry, or action learning), we have simply used the term clinical action research as a shorthand instead of the more unwieldy 'action research taking place in clinical settings'. The predominant differences between clinical action research and, for example, educational action research conducted in controlled settings in education institutions lies in the nature of culture, the context and collaboration. The attitudes, values, goals, and practices that characterise healthcare organisations, the dynamic clinical context, the clinical action researcher/facilitator and co-researchers as both autonomous practitioners and multidisciplinary team members, all have an impact on a patient-centred action research project. The fundamental principles of action research remain the same (as for other disciplines), but the conduct of action research in diverse hospital and community healthcare settings, including care homes, with people with a range of often complex needs, and with multidisciplinary colleagues, requires a different focus for consideration. As in many healthcare policy documents and healthcare books, we have used a number of terms for 'patient', including service user, client, consumer and participant in care.

This book has been written for readers at different stages of their 'journey' as action researchers: some will be experienced in the field and will be looking for new insights and ideas about how to conduct their next projects, supported by the increasing action research literature; other readers will be at the novice end of the spectrum and looking for ideas about how best to start, plan and manage their clinical action research projects. It is obviously a challenging task addressing the different needs of interested readers. We hope that we have offered a rich mixture of theoretical material on the roots and antecedents of action research, on the different 'varieties' or nuanced approaches to the design and conduct of action research, as well as examples from our own and others' work which shed light on interesting and difficult questions that action researchers often face in clinical settings. In this book issues of data collection and analysis are considered, but we believe that it is also important for action researchers to consult and use major sources from established authors in their fields, in detail and with a level of critical analysis that, due to chapter length restrictions, we are unable to supply in this text. We have endeavoured to maintain a writing style that is reasonably closely aligned, but as the chapters have been written by three authors, some differences in style and emphasis are inevitable. We also recognise the increasing use of creative writing, including poetic expression, in practitioner research. It is likely that readers will want to dip into chapters that they will find useful on their action research journey as well as reading the book through from the first chapter to the last.

The book contains several features that will help the reader to understand, assimilate and make use of the content. Each chapter opens with several clear objectives which outline what the reader can gain from the chapter, with a summary at the end of the chapter showing briefly how the objectives have been addressed. In addition, each chapter has a number of reflective activities which enable the reader to engage with the material and to understand and think through how it is directly relevant to their own setting. Some chapters include further reading and other resources such as websites. Terminology is explained in the text and there is also a Glossary at the end of the book.

The text is divided into four parts, these being:

- Section 1: What is action research?
- Section 2: Why choose action research?
- Section 3: Conducting action research in clinical practice
- Section 4: Disseminating and evaluating clinical action research projects

In Section 1: What is action research? Chapter 1 is called Foundations of Action Research and because it is important to understand the foundations of action research and to explore different approaches to action research, we examine some of the philosophical issues underpinning action research and outline the work of early theorists, including Kurt Lewin and the influence of the critical theorists as well as more recent aspects of action research design. In Chapter 2: Discussion, Debate and Controversy Surrounding Action Research, we argue that criticism of action research often centres on its perceived subjectivity and potential for bias due to the proximity of researchers and participants, but that it can instead be seen as a 'new **paradigm**' approach which does not need to subscribe to its critics' demands for a traditional approach to research rigour. Various issues are discussed concerning 'scientific' research standards and action research.

Section 2 addresses the question Why Choose Action Research? Chapter 3 is called Action Research, Nursing and Healthcare, and in it we explore some of the underpinning ideas concerning the application of action research to nursing and healthcare practice. We argue that action research is recognised as a sustainable force for change among diverse communities in global healthcare settings.

Chapter 4 is Clinical Action Research to Advance Patient Care, and here we argue that action research is suited to healthcare settings. We explore the role of the clinical action researcher in advancing practice-based research and development, looking particularly at the clinical context and how organisational culture impacts on a project.

In Section 3, Conducting Action Research in Clinical Practice, Chapter 5 is called Developing One's Own Professional Practice and reflects on how action research can form an integral part of developing one's own practice. Using the specific example of the action research that one of us (JW) undertook as a Consultant Nurse for Older People, it illustrates how working collaboratively with others can be complex, challenging and rewarding. We move on from the substantive example in Chapter 5 to examine some more theoretical material, as well as other examples. In Chapter 6, Collaborative Working in Clinical Settings, we explore some theoretical issues concerning collaboration, facilitation and team working, and emphasise the need for greater clinical academic linkage. Chapter 7, Ethical Considerations, examines the ethical implications of engaging in collaborative action research in clinical settings, identifies the challenges of ethical approval for user engagement and explores practical approaches for ethical approval in the NHS and in Universities.

In Section 4: Disseminating and Evaluating Clinical Action Research Projects, we consider, in separate chapters, how to write up studies, present them to different audiences, and also highlight some of the criteria that have been used to evaluate action research studies. Chapter 8: Writing Clinical Action Research Studies examines what to write and how to convey action research projects in different ways. It focuses on the key areas to address in the writing of action research studies and the differences between internal report writing, writing for a higher degree and writing articles for publication in academic and peer-reviewed 'popular' journals. We also consider the challenges, criticism and creativity that exist in writing up action research studies. Chapter 9: Presenting Clinical Action Research Studies to Mixed Audiences has some important points about getting your message across in different settings, specifically knowing your audience, the requirements of effective presentation and new media and the mass media. The last chapter of Section 4 is Chapter 10: Evaluating the Quality of Action Research Projects, in which we argue that action researchers, funding bodies, ethics committees, participants and readers need a shared understanding of how to evaluate the quality of action research proposals, projects and written reports. We provide some ideas and examine some tools which can be useful in doing that.

The last chapter of the book provides some concluding material, and we have called it Looking to the Future because as well as summarising what we have achieved in the book it also looks at how action research might undergo further growth in the UK as a result of policy changes and developments and the need for continuous development of clinical practice. We also take a global perspective by examining some of the studies that have been undertaken since 2000 and published in selected journals. Our concluding remarks indicate that we see a growing use of action research in healthcare settings as practitioners, researchers and academics seek to work together to affect beneficial change in clinical practice settings.

We are grateful to our critical reviewers, Professor David Coghlan and Dr Angela Grainger, for their insightful feedback on many of the following chapters. We are also grateful to Professor Brendan McCormack for supporting the book proposal, and to the team at SAGE for their constructive comments and advice at all stages of the process.

**Graham R Williamson, Loretta Bellman
and Jonathan Webster**

SECTION 1

WHAT IS ACTION RESEARCH?

1

FOUNDATIONS OF ACTION RESEARCH

Graham R Williamson

It is important to understand the foundations of action research and to explore different approaches to action research as there are subtle differences of emphasis and suitability for different situations.

Chapter objectives

This chapter will examine:

- some of the philosophical issues underpinning action research and outline the work of early theorists, including Kurt Lewin's pioneering work and the influence of critical theory
- some of the key theoretical and interrelated aspects of action research, including:
    - human inquiry, cooperative inquiry and action science/action inquiry
    - participatory action research
    - action research and **feminsim**
    - appreciative inquiry

Introduction

Simply put, action research is a process by which change is achieved and new knowledge about a situation is generated. These two objectives go hand-in-hand to a greater or lesser degree in most action research studies: it is difficult to change a situation without working to understand it more fully, and in trying better to understand things, the possibilities for change often emerge.

Coghlan and Brannick (2010) outline four broad characteristics of action research. These are:

1 Action research is about research *in* action rather than *about* action. Thus a 'scientific' process of inquiry is used in social settings to link important issues with those who experience them.
2 It is a collaborative, **democratic** process, meaning that there is active participation of those who experience the situation in working towards solutions. This is distinct from traditional research approaches, both quantitative and qualitative, where research participants are subjects rather than collaborators.
3 Action and knowledge are joined so that change occurs while there is a simultaneous process of knowledge generation.
4 It is a sequence of events and an approach to problem solving which contributes to knowledge and understanding.

Box 1.1

This is a lengthy quote, which illustrates the challenge of being able clearly to define AR! For Waterman et al. (2001: iii), action research is

> a period of inquiry that describes, interprets and explains social situations while executing a change intervention aimed at improvement and involvement. It is problem-focused, context-specific and future-oriented...founded on partnership...educative and empowering. ... Knowledge may be advanced through reflection and research, and qualitative and quantitative research methods may be employed to collect data.

Action research has been described (Reason and Bradbury 2006) as a 'new **paradigm**' in its focusing of research on participation and change. Research approaches are frequently discussed as coming from qualitative or quantitative **paradigms**, and although there is discussion and debate in the methodological literature concerning the underpinning theoretical positions each occupies, they are still frequently discussed as quite different ways of thinking about and doing research (there is more on this in Chapter 2). Quantitative research seeks to demonstrate an external reality through manipulation and control of variables and is based on a tradition of objectivity and **positivism.** This is frequently contrasted with qualitative research, which comes from a **hermeneutic** or **interpretivist paradigm**, in which the ability of human beings to construct and understand their lives is emphasised, and there is no fixed external reality (these arguments are more fully explored in Chapter 2). While some argue that this qualitative/quantitative dichotomy is a false one

(Morrow and Brown 1994), it is clear that action research fits fully with neither of these traditions, but has features of each, in that a process of change is applied to social life, whereas the reflexive nature of individuals and groups within any setting is also emphasised. This can be radical as it challenges traditional research approaches, existing forms of social organisation in the workplace and in society (Coghlan and Brannick 2010), and is described as **democratic** and participatory.

Action research has been quite recently adopted by healthcare professionals seeking to develop aspects of their practice and that of their organisations. It is not simply a 'tool' for practice development or change management; it has a long history in many sectors, and roots and a philosophical tradition which, arguably, go back to the early part of the twentieth century.

Philosophical issues and action research

The philosophical issues encompass the extent to which participation and change can be fostered in action research, and it is important to consider these because they provide a different emphasis and intention from traditional research approaches. A foundation stone for action research appears to lie in the political philosophy of the critical theorists.

Critical theory

Originally a term associated with the Marxist-oriented Frankfurt Institute for Social Research, which was founded in Germany in 1923, 'critical theory' is now taken to mean an approach to social sciences that offers a critique of existing social relations as well as a perspective on how things should be changed, developed or improved. The original Frankfurt School included 'famous names' from the broad field of sociology and psychology, such as Horkheimer, Adorno, Marcuse and Fromm, many of whom moved to Columbia University in the USA in the 1930s to avoid Nazism. A 'second generation', including figures such as Offe, and Habermas, was influential in the 1960s and beyond, with Marcuse in particular influencing **democratic** and political reforms in favour of the 'new social movements', which sought greater freedoms for groups such as women, ethnic minorities and followers of single-issue politics such as the Green movement (Bronner and Kellner 1989).

Critical theory is seen as an 'antidote' to the quantitative or '**positivist**' tradition in research, which is argued to be uncritical, and therefore unlikely to generate social change (Bronner and Kellner 1989). The underlying premise of critical theory is concerned with human happiness and that this can be attained only by transforming all aspects of social life (Marcuse 1989). Critical theorists' focus is on the issue of domination: how some groups in society control all aspects of the lives of others, and thus inhibit those in oppressed groups from realising their full potential. Following Marx, critical theorists argue that economic power and class are the roots of oppression and the crucial factor is changing these existing power relations. Some critical theorists thus have an interest in beneficial change, or 'transformative praxis' (Morrow and Brown 1994: 27; although it is not the case that all critical theorists unambiguously associate 'critical theory' and a drive towards 'praxis') and their work is frequently described as being concerned with **emancipation** (Kellner 1989).

••• REFLECTIVE ACTIVITY 1.1 •••

1 What is your understanding of the term 'praxis'?
2 What is the additional meaning implied by adding 'transformative' to make 'transformative praxis'?
3 How would you define the concept of '**emancipation**'?

••• ANSWERS •••

1 Praxis means a process by which a theory or skill is applied to the real world. It also has a political meaning: to change social relations, with connotations of theory and practice informing each other as change occurs. It can also mean 'making visible' and acting upon one's values.
2 While different authors use the term differently, it seems as if adding the term 'transformative' implies the intention on the part of authors to change aspects of social life in conjunction with those with whom they are interacting. There is an explicit 'looking forward' to the achievement of greater equality, or social justice, or overturning of exploitative power relations. 'Transformative praxis' thus has a more overtly political tone than using the term 'praxis' alone.
3 **Emancipation** means to become free or be set free. In the context of critical theory, **emancipation** can mean freedom from oppression or exploitation, in terms of economic power, gender relations or ethnicity.

Habermas's critical social science

The work of Habermas may be unfamiliar to you but it can provide a philosophical basis for change in contemporary society. Habermas (1981) identifies three **knowledge-constitutive paradigms**, underpinning what he calls the 'empirical–analytical', the 'historical–**hermeneutic**' and the 'critical' sciences. The empirical–analytical sciences' base is technical control of the natural world. This instrumental knowledge generates rules, which the **Natural sciences** use for explanation and prediction (Carr and Kemmis 1986), for example as in quantitative research. The historical–**hermeneutic** sciences owe their genesis to the need for effective communication in contemporary societies, both between individuals and traditions and between different traditions. Methods in the historical–**hermeneutic** sciences are interpretive and 'practical', allowing people to understand their social worlds and their histories (Carr and Kemmis 1986), as for example in qualitative research; where communication breaks down, interaction becomes problematic. However, it would appear that only the 'critical' sciences offer the potential for transcending the constraints of the former two sciences, to grasp at **emancipation**: action research is taken as an example of a research technique from the critical sciences (Morrow and Brown 1994). This **emancipation** does not, for Habermas, preclude using either empirical–analytical, or historical–**hermeneutic** methods, but the potential for self-reflection is implicitly critical, challenging dysfunctional and oppressive structures whether they are political, economic, social or organisational. Thus an ethical dimension can be re-introduced into contemporary social life (Carr and Kemmis 1986), and praxis can be established as a guiding principle in social science research.

However, identifying and establishing praxis as a central tenet of contemporary life is problematic, not least because there may be many interpretations of what challenges there should be, how praxis can be identified and sustained, and what constitutes a new ethical dimension. For Carr and Kemmis (1986) , Habermas's critical social science cannot reconcile the need for praxis with the need to meet the 'scientific' **positivist** notions of rigour which society has come to expect in research. Even so, Habermas shows that social science can claim **validity** based on shared understanding rather than the laws of the **natural sciences**, meaning that consensus about the **validity** of a discourse is not subject to the measurement of objective criteria but is a **democratic** event, as people participate equally in what he refers to as the 'ideal speech act'. This discourse involves four **validity** claims: (1) that what is said is *true*;(2) that the utterance is *comprehensible*;(3) that the speaker is *sincere*; and (4) that it is *right* for the speaker to be speaking.

For social scientists, Habermas implicitly calls for change-centred action, as critical social science is about the development of theory, the organisation of learning processes and the organisation of action: political 'doing', aimed at **emancipation**. In this manner, social scientists can facilitate 'communicative action', which tests the accuracy, sincerity and rightness of social processes, including organisational life. For Habermas, social life in contemporary society has been appropriated by purposive-rational action and functional reason, meaning that mutual understanding and consensus are virtually suspended in modern organisational life: people are divided and fragmented by the social relations of bureaucracy and expert systems (Kemmis 1996); they simply get on with the job but this is not cost-free, causing crises borne by individuals and systems. As work roles become increasingly elaborate and differentiated, communities are increasingly difficult to sustain, and there is an 'uncoupling' of system and **lifeworld** (see below) for those who inhabit them (Habermas 1987).

Habermas and action research

For Kemmis (2006), action researchers engage with the Habermas thesis, as they explicitly act on three kinds of **lifeworld processes**. These are: (1) the process of individuation-socialisation, by which participants' identities are formed; (2) social integration, forming and developing social relations; and (3) cultural reproduction, by which shared cultures and discourses are developed. Moreover, action researchers investigate and seek to change the ways in which participants are enmeshed in systems functioning. Kemmis (2006) argues that action research (AR) is an opportunity to create communicative action in participants as it illustrates and improves the alienating nature of contemporary organisations by its imperative to participate.

However, the action research movement predated Habermas by many years, and so Habermas provides retrospectively a philosophical background for methodologies advocated by action researchers (Kemmis and McTaggart 1990). Also, it is worth reflecting that although Habermas (1981) argues that contemporary societies should look critically at the over-arching dominance of **natural science** understanding, it is here that a key question arises for critical theory and similarly for action research, that is: Whose **emancipation** are we talking about? In critical theory there is an assumption that the 'common good' will appear from collective action, but this is by no means certain as what is good for one group or individual is not necessarily good for others, and the will of the majority is not necessarily clearly expressed or unconditionally good. Action researchers must be clear that they themselves do not simply impose the majority will on others as this would be oppressive.

The diversity of action research

Kurt Lewin's pioneering work

Kurt Lewin is frequently credited with pioneering early AR work (Dickens and Watkins 1999; McNiff 1988), and with coining the term 'action research' (Carr and Kemmis 1986; Greenwood and Levin 1998), although there is debate about the extent to which he inherited the idea from others (McNiff and Whitehead 2002). Lewin criticised his contemporaries' disconnected academic research, saying 'research that produces nothing but books will not suffice' (Lewin 1946: 35). He was convinced that social scientists should develop and apply techniques to equip groups with the ability to change aspects of their social or organisational lives for themselves (McNiff 1988). He conceptualised action research as a spiral methodology involving discrete phases (Lewin 1946):

- first, a planning or fact-finding phase, beginning with a general idea following extended 'diagnosis', and next,
- the implementation or execution of the plan, with this 'experimental' phase followed by further fact finding to evaluate the results of the action.

Lewin's (1946) work on 'minority problems describes a four-step cycle of action research (Figure 1.1), and he advocates repeated turns around the cycle so that the experience gained in the evaluation phase can be reapplied to the experimental phase.

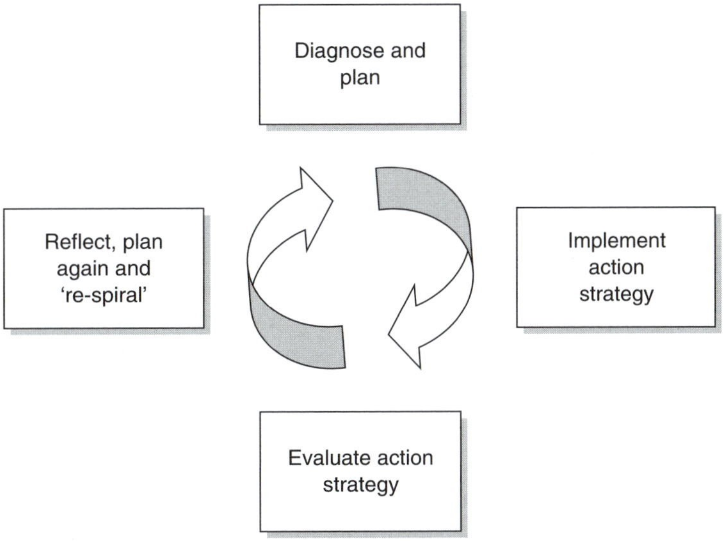

Figure 1.1 Action research spiral framework (adapted from Lewin 1946)

However, a critical evaluation of this spiral framework indicates that it has certain weaknesses (Winter and Munn-Giddings 2001).

1 It appears to oversimplify a complex iterative process, suggesting that the overall 'goal' in AR remains fixed when this is frequently not the case.
2 The emphasis on repeated spirals implies that AR must have a long time scale when this need not be the case.
3 AR seems difficult to distinguish from everyday interaction with colleagues, and so a criticism is whether or not AR really is a 'research' methodology.

Winter and Munn-Giddings (2001) continue by saying that AR is actually an ideal methodology for changing workplace practice, and the emphasis on reflection means that new knowledge and understanding are generated.

In work aimed at changing eating habits, Lewin (1966) demonstrated the relative efficacy of group decision-making processes compared to experts' exhortations by setting up a series of 'experiments' using his spiral AR methodology. In a study which aimed to alter mothers' preferences for certain foods, he examined whether his female participants would serve orange juice, cod liver oil, and fresh and evaporated milk to their families. He found that they were much more likely to introduce these 'new' foods when involved in a group decision-making process as opposed to receiving only a health education lecture. He was able to show that he could change elements of a pre-existing social system.

Although Lewin discusses 'experimentation' as predictive of participants' behaviour and sees the social system as relatively fixed following his 'intervention', unlike in a traditional scientific **paradigm**, results are studied in order to adjust the strategy and to refine it. There are no tightly set limits or controls on the 'experimentation', and the action researcher approaches the participants in their 'natural' state (Dickens and Watkins 1999).

Lewin's work was the building block for today's AR movement, setting the stage for a methodology that produces knowledge for the solution of real-world problems. He developed a new role for the researcher, and redefined criteria for judging the inquiry process. He also 'relocated' researchers, so that instead of disconnected observation, participation and concrete problem solving are central to their role. This was a radical departure from previous 'command and control' strategies intended to regulate workers' lives (Greenwood and Levin 1998), meaning that, rather than simply diffusing or disseminating new ideas in academic journals, action researchers are instrumental in the implementation of solutions to the problems they help to identify (Sitzia 2001).

Varieties of action research

Although in the following discussion the major strands of AR are treated distinctly, they are by no means so distinct, and there is a considerable overlapping and sharing of ideas, despite a somewhat different emphasis. These slightly different perspectives are included so that readers can get a flavour of the AR work that has taken place.

Human inquiry, cooperative inquiry and action science/action inquiry

Human inquiry, cooperative inquiry and action science/action inquiry are closely related AR strands (Greenwood and Levin 1998). The central emphasis is on human experience and engagement, as distinct from today's perceived alienated living.

Human inquiry

For Reason, AR is a philosophical movement with an approach to living as much as a research approach, and it is not only about the search for truth, but should 'heal' (Reason 1994a: 10) the alienation of modern existence. Critics may see this as a call for bias, but this is false as, he argues, human beings are fundamentally located in the world, not abstracted from it. **Positivistic** principles bring a detrimental loss of relationships with other people, but this can be overcome by participation. This is a **dialectical** process of change where tension and contradiction drive forward the evolution of a future participatory human consciousness.

Cooperative inquiry

Cooperative inquiry is a variant of AR which is about finding ways of working with people who have similar concerns in order to understand the shared aspects of their worlds and to learn how to act to change things for the better (Heron and Reason 2006). Its micro-political format encourages individuals and groups to cooperate against controlling authoritarian processes (Heron 2001), and it has roots in humanistic psychology. Cooperative inquiry seeks 'authentic communication', for which orthodox social science methodology is inadequate as it excludes human beings from decision-making processes in research. In cooperative inquiry, those involved should be reciprocating co-researchers, reflecting the essential self-determining character of human beings. It takes place in four phases of action and reflection, which rely on certain ideas about the nature of knowledge. These are:

- that co-researchers identify research propositions based on their experience, and identify procedures to observe and record their experience (propositional knowledge);
- that these procedures are applied to their everyday life and work, searching for nuisances and subtleties in the work (practical knowing);
- that new insights arise for the researchers as a result of their engagement in the project, developing an openness that allows them to bracket off personal beliefs to see the issues in a new way (experiential knowledge);
- that after a time in phase three, co-researchers return to their original propositions, reconsider and modify them in the light of experience, reformulating and reframing the question. This phase involves returning with a critical perspective to co-researchers' propositional knowledge (Reason, 1994b) (see Figure 1.2).

Critical examination of Figure 1.2 indicates how action research links insights from participants' real-world experience with a drive to change social situations in a similar fashion to that identified by Lewin (1946) and presented in Figure 1.1 (Reason (1994b) and Heron and Reason (2006)). What neither figure shows is how this circular two-dimensional representation is

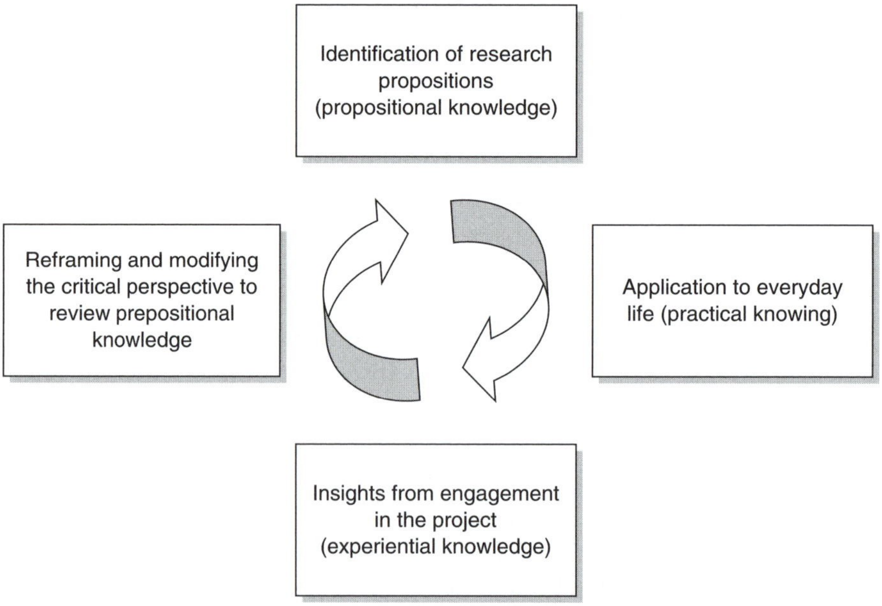

Figure 1.2 Four-phase spiral of action and reflection (adapted from Reason 1994b and Heron and Reason 2006)

actually a three-dimensional spiral in which action researchers can reflect on and revisit their understanding with new insights gained from the project.

Action inquiry and action science

In action inquiry and action science, there is an emphasis on developing effective action to transform organisations, producing greater effectiveness and justice (Reason 1994b). Central to action science are two cognitive theories of action. These are espoused theories, which individuals claim to use, and theories-in-use, which can be inferred from actions (Argyris and Schön 1974). These may be consistent or inconsistent, and the actor may or may not be aware of any inconsistency. In organisations, there are two models of action relating to cognitive theories-in-use. Model I is a defensive and self-protective theory, and Model II encourages free choice and open inquiry (Argyris and Schön 1974; Reason 1994b; Coghlan and Brannick 2010). Overcoming organisational defensiveness is a key element in action science to enable personal learning and practice development.

In action inquiry, organisations create structures to enable learning to take place so that individuals can become self-reflective about their work practices (Reason 1994b). For Torbert (2006), all action is a form of inquiry. Individuals and organisations need to go beyond the single-loop nature of learning from the impact and consequences of immediate actions only, to the more powerful double-loop reconstruction of personal and professional life strategies. However, it can be difficult to be self-reflective, and traditional social science research does not offer a means for doing this. Therefore, action inquiry is required to study both the 'outside' of the external universe as well as the 'inside' of 'territories of experience' (Torbert 2006: 208). There are four of these, which Torbert calls:

- visioning, which is a planning function looking to the future;
- strategising, which is developing ways of moving forward;
- performing, which is about carrying out the strategies; and
- assessing, which is about deciding on successes, failures and future actions.

Thus there is an emphasis on cognitive transformations in the individual, located in a wider organisational context (Greenwood and Levin 1998).

Participatory action research

Participatory action research (PAR) emphasises the emancipatory potential inherent in AR methodology, involving a transformation of some aspect of a community's situation or structures. It focuses on issues of power, the exclusion of the powerless from decision-making and how they can be included (Coghlan and Brannick 2010), and harnesses the lived experience of oppressed groups (Reason 1994b). It has an explicitly critical stance, which paradoxically seeks to transform the wider social order but is usually most effective in local situations (Healy 2001).

For Koch and Kralik (2006), there is an explicitly transformative agenda in their PAR work (examples of their work are discussed in Chapter 3), one that seeks to liberate, empower and reform situations as well as give substance to the voices of participants, who may previously have been excluded and marginalised. Their overriding concern is with 'making a difference' and their methodological approach is informed by critical theory and feminist thought. Thus PAR is a form of action directed towards social change which also includes a strong element of consciousness-raising: enabling participants to see how they may unwittingly contribute to their own oppression through discussion and reflection, and helping them to develop ways of overcoming it. This can be an explicitly political purpose where the intention is to restore power to oppressed groups. PAR is intended to go beyond abstracted 'scientific' methodology and narrowly focused Lewin-type AR to lay foundations for change in social conditions which communities themselves fashion. It is critical of ineffective research techniques, exhibits a radical social conscience, and demands **democratic** participation to find better scientific, technical and social ways to improve living conditions (Fals Borda 2006). In healthcare settings, PAR may not be so overtly political but is more concerned with changing practices and understanding of needs; while change is central, generating new knowledge is also an important consideration.

In PAR, researchers and participants systematically work in cycles to explore issues that have an impact on the lives of participants (Koch and Kralik 2006). A simple, three-stage cyclical approach of 'Look, Think and Act' (which Koch and Kralik adapted from Stringer's 1999 work; see Figure 1.3) gives structure as well as flexibility to the work, as it enables researchers and participants to focus on a particular area, reflect on and discuss its characteristics, and then reconstruct these experiences and decide courses of action.

This structure is not rigid or prescriptive and moves along according to the needs and requirements of participants. Research meetings may include Looking, Thinking and Action planning all together or may simply focus on one element. In the Looking phase, a picture is created of the issue in question. In the Think phase, there is a focus on interpreting and explaining things. In the Act phase, action is taken to resolve issues and this action is evaluated. Frequently, more than one cycle is undertaken.

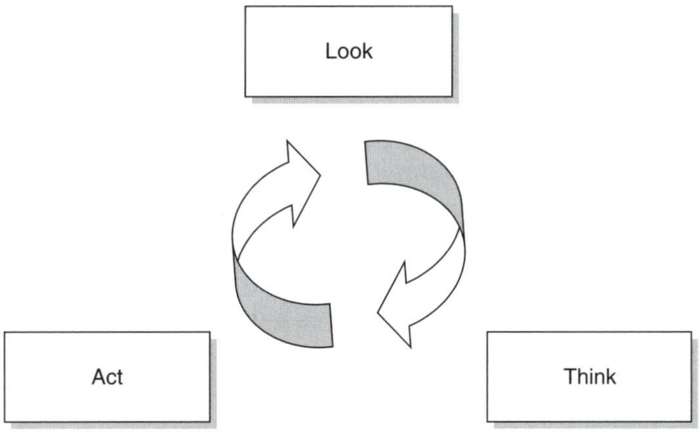

Figure 1.3 PAR cycles 'Look, Think and Act' (adapted from Koch and Kralik 2006: 28)

PAR is a community-based approach in that a community is constructed and maintained in which the researchers and participants are considered to be on an equal level, with the premise that a social situation or organisation ought to change for the better to enhance the lives of its members. Thus (drawing on Stringer's 1999 work) Koch and Kralik (2006; Figure 1.3) describe PAR as:

- **democratic**,
- equitable,
- liberating, and
- life-enhancing.

Critical examination of Koch and Kralik's (2006) framework indicates that, similar to Lewin's (1946) spiral, it would appear to simplify too much what Koch and Kralik (2006) themselves identify as flexible and complex action research processes, and again does not acknowledge fully the spiral nature of action research.

• • • REFLECTIVE ACTIVITY 1.2 • • •

- Identify an area from work life with which you are not content. Explain why you not are content. Are there elements of power and powerlessness in what you identify?

- Using a three-stage PAR process of Look, Think and Act, write down your thoughts on what the issue is and how you might change the situation.
    - Look: identify the issue.
    - Think: reflect on its nature and characteristics. You are thinking through this alone, but as you will need colleagues and friends, users and carers to help and support you, reflect on who would be good co-researchers and participants. You will no doubt find that working with others on this gives a deeper understanding of the situation, a greater sense of purpose, an element of camaraderie and ownership of the project which would be of benefit to you all.
    - Act: how might you change things and how would you know you have been successful? Who would be the key people you would need to convince and what mechanisms and resources would you use to do so?

As this is a personal activity, no suggestions for answers have been included. However, if you were to use this as a project framework, can you see how identifying new knowledge in the Look and Think phases could quickly become change-focused action in the Act phase? (See Chapter 4 for a more detailed presentation about using AR to develop clinical care.)

Action research and feminsim

Feminist research is more than simply research done by women for/or with women; rather, it is an approach that makes its central concerns the needs of women and improving their lives, as well as breaking down the barriers between researcher and participants. For some authors, there is an explicitly critical dimension in that existing power relations between men and women are unequal and men's domination of society is oppressive to women (Webb 1993).

Several feminist writers have seen the emancipatory potential of AR. Greenwood and Levin (1998) outline how the feminist agenda and PAR overlap: suspicion or inappropriateness of **positivism**; analysis of power relations; respect for the knowledge of the 'silenced'; interest in transforming and emancipating praxis. These ideas should replace traditional research approaches in the social sciences, which are currently in turmoil as new **paradigms** replace old certainties in society and well as in research (Lather 1991). **Feminism** and AR are not competing frameworks but share a critical perspective that makes them allies as, for Lather (1988) and Piran (2001), **feminism** has helped create a space where a debate about power and the production of knowledge can be held. Feminist research, then, is about both change and developing new knowledge, and thus shares similar aims to AR, albeit with the intention of uncovering and redressing the distorted power relations that exist between men and women.

Maguire (2006) argues that **feminism** has informed AR and helped create the conditions for its success because of the feminist critique of abstract knowledge. Winter and Munn-Giddings (2001) and Meyer (1993) note that both AR and feminist research value experiential knowledge and the importance of doing research *with* rather than *on* participants. Pioneering feminist work such as Oakley's (1981) redefined interviewing by relocating it away from traditional 'scientific' and detached approaches, focusing instead on women's shared identity, usable findings and a more open and participative process. 'Standpoint', meaning the position from which issues are viewed, is important. Thus women will have a very different perspective on, for example, childbirth, than a man ever can, and this shared understanding can and should inform their research. This applies in AR in that proximity and shared understanding with participants is a goal, and this is likely to be enhanced if a researcher shares membership of a particular group. Arguably, this is particularly important in research in healthcare, where a whole dimension of experience is potentially lost because subjects are frequently women, and policy-makers and researchers are often men.

AR and feminist research point in the same direction: to uncover, analyse and improve the position of disadvantaged groups within society by hearing their hidden voices (Winter and Munn-Giddings 2001). Feminists and action researchers should collaborate, as both make possible research avoiding the temptation for academics to speak for individuals, instead allowing them to use their own skills and voices to develop an understanding of their lives (Hollingsworth 1997). This is particularly important in practice settings where women predominate, such as in teaching, social work and nursing. Hollingsworth (1997) notes that AR is inherently emancipatory because it challenges existing masculine forms of authority and knowledge, arguing that one measure of success in feminist AR is the extent to which it is transformational. This is echoed by Koch and Kralik (2006) and Weiner (2004), who see PAR as offering genuinely emancipatory potential for feminists, arguing that PAR offers the ability for women to realise their potential by overcoming masculine domination, and so gender relations are their central focus. Koch and Kralik (2006) further identify five issues of importance when using PAR for feminist research. These are as follows:

- The researcher's position. Here, the aim is a non-hierarchical and reflexive approach to research that may challenge the researcher as well as the participants, but the researcher must understand that the research is owned by the participants, that their voices must emerge, and that this can be very powerful.

- Participation and action. Here, Koch and Kralik (2006) argue that, as feminist researchers, they experience close connections with their participants. This leads to genuine mutuality in the production of data – they are all co-participants rather than 'researchers and researched'.
- Disclosure of experiences. This means that telling the story is incredibly important and therapeutic for participants, and that in the telling new meaning occurs as people's experiences are voiced and receive affirmation from others.
- Consciousness-raising. As feminist research aims to raise consciousness of women's oppressed position in society with participants and with those in the wider arena, specifically with participants, the intention is to narrow the gap between them and encourage reciprocity through reflexive understanding.
- Feminist PAR with non-feminist women. Feminist conceptions of power may not be helpful to those without a feminist understanding, so researchers' conceptions may dominate the research agenda when they are not explicitly wanted by non-feminist participants, and thus researchers can be accused of leading participants down paths of discussion to suit their own agenda. Sensitivity and balance are therefore always required in feminist PAR.

Griffiths (1994) aligns herself with the critical theory perspective, saying that AR is political for individual participants and can have a wider political impact, but also argues that AR should rightly begin with the personal. She argues that AR, and writing about AR, are essentially autobiographical acts. Journals or diaries form part of the 'tool-kit'. This gives a powerful critique of abstract 'masculinist' knowledge, which seeks distance and abstraction from reality. Autobiographical writing opens the door for a subjective conscience, and this enables the 'hidden' voices of women to become heard in a way not previously possible. This is empowering and is part of a new theorising of 'difference', or gender inequality. There is emancipatory potential for men as well as women because mutual and inclusive gender relations are only possible if both genders' voices are heard. AR thus has a wider political significance because as a methodology it can uncover women's voices, particularly in 'hidden' occupations like teaching and nursing. However, the relationship between AR and **feminism** remains 'uneven ground' (Maguire 2006), as action researchers have been slow to acknowledge and develop the links. Weiner (2004) goes further, arguing that linking critical theory and action research misses the potential to explicitly link change through action research with a feminist emancipatory agenda.

Appreciative inquiry

A change process known as appreciative inquiry (AI) uses elements of AR. AI was developed in his doctoral studies by David Cooperrider in the 1980s. When he interviewed Cleveland Clinic clinical staff about their successes and failures, he found the success stories powerful and focused on them. His findings had a huge impact on the Clinic and its board, who requested that he use them throughout the organisation (Seel 2008). AI focuses on the need for change, but is based on taking a positive approach, so rather than focusing on what is wrong, AI results in the synergy and commitment of individuals and departments by seeking to discover the best possible outcomes and working towards them, seeing the glass as half full rather than half empty (Lewis and Van Tiem 2004). As Cooperrider (2008) puts it, AI turns change management on its head, as instead of expecting another survey of low morale to change the workplace culture, what is required is an awareness of high 'commitment work systems', which can occur by tapping into how workers experience the best aspects of their own working lives. Rather than a small group of managers doing the work and rolling out the findings, if strategic change is required, the number of participants should be hundreds, even thousands of employees at once, in the same place, cooperating to bring about real organisational change.

A '4-D cycle of discovery' is utilised (see Figure 1.4): discovery, dream, design and destiny. This is not a fixed or prescriptive framework, but rather a map of a journey of engagement between participants and organisational change (Moore 2008). The process begins with an appreciative interview and focuses participants' energies towards identifying an answer to the question 'What do you really want?' It is thus concerned with consolidating a vision of a better future into achievable directions. This is a wholly positive endeavour, with an unconditionally positive question framed for participants (Cooperrider et al. 2005). AI is based on five principles (Cooperrider and Whitney 2005). These are:

1 The constructionist principle. This states that individuals are continually negotiating, communicating and interacting with those around them, and that this interaction builds organisational change. Knowledge thus has a communal basis. The function of AI is to chart future success based on previous achievements, rather than simply solve problems.
2 The simultaneity principle. This states that inquiry and change are intertwined. These are reflected in the questions asked, and these questions are an important factor in the direction in which change occurs.
3 The poetic principle. This holds that organisations are not closed machines but open, human activities. The past, present and future are

constantly open to change from the different interpretations placed in them by different people, in the same way that poetry or literature is interpreted differently by different people.

4 The anticipatory principle. Positive images of the future lead to positive transitions. What organisations focus on is what they get, so a positive focus on beneficial change is more likely to be successful than a continual focus on short-term problem-solving.
5 The positive principle. The more positive and uplifting, the more a sense of shared understanding and camaraderie are generated by AI, the more likely successful and long-lasting change will be.

Critical appraisal of Figure 1.4 suggests that it too has an emphasis on a singular turn of the circle, rather than an evolutionary spiral. However, this may make it suitable for visionary or transformative events in clearly defined contexts.

In the Discovery phase, the emphasis is not on identifying problems, but is about listening to and understanding what individuals believe to be the positive aspects of working in the organisation, what they consider to work well, and their successes. As Lewis and Van Tiem (2004: 21) state, '[t]elling their stories and having witnesses is an exceptionally transforming experience' for individuals and ultimately organisations. In the Dream phase, the drive is to promote a vision of excellence so that groups of workers are encouraged to dream about what the organisation might be like if the excellence they identify in the Discovery phase were, in fact, their routine practice. In the Design phase, groups of participants work out how to change the

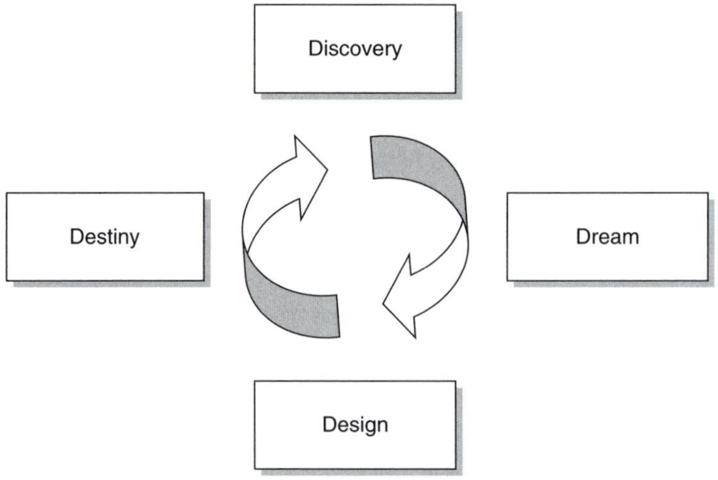

Figure 1.4 Appreciative inquiry 4-D cycle (adapted from Moore 2008)

organisation for the better to make their dreams for it come true, looking at the specifics of how to get things done. The Destiny (or Deliver) phase is where organisational cultures and structures are actually changed. Further work should also take place using further 4-D cycles.

This positive emphasis and imagery is very powerful. Even the most profoundly negative elements of a workplace can be accommodated by good facilitation (see Chapter 6), which can work to turn the negatives into positives: using empathy and good listening skills, participants can be induced to outline how things *should* have been and thus how they *might* be (Seel 2008). AI thus encourages a collaborative approach between members of different organisational departments, and potentially between other organisations, which might otherwise find themselves in opposition or working towards conflicting goals. By focusing on the positive aspects of social life, AI reduces defensiveness and encourages discussion and collaboration (Reed et al. 2002).

For Oliver (2005), AI is uncritical in the sense that it does not challenge existing power relations, and she seeks to reframe it as *critical appreciative inquiry*. This should acknowledge power relations and encourage a less hierarchical approach than is the norm in organisations, and this understanding can be beneficial for management practice.

In healthcare, AI has been used to improve care for patients and clients. For example, Guilar and Start (2001) used AI for South Southwark Primary Care Group to improve diabetes care with six general practices in London. Patients and professionals including nurses and doctors attended. The workshop focused on the question 'How can we enable people with diabetes to manage their diabetes as well as possible?' This question focused on positive aspects, hoping to turn them into reality. Their interviews used a script full of positive potential.

Box 1.2

1. Talk about a particular incident when you enabled someone to manage their diabetes more effectively.
2. What do you think you/your organisation/the service does really well when managing diabetes?
3. If overnight a miracle happened and the diabetes service you and your practice/unit provided was exactly how you would like it to be:
   a. What would be the same?
   b. What would be different?

Guilar and Start's (2001) diabetes care interview script. Adapted from Guilar and Start (2001: 85)

Including patients as participants was extremely valuable, as they offered useful insights when asked 'What has been really helpful in managing your diabetes care?' The whole project enabled real change to take place in the management of diabetes care in this area of London, and three new services were established as a result (Guilar and Start 2001). These were:

- A GP/Practice Nurse Diabetic Forum for collaboration between the community staff and the consultant diabetologists.
- A Diabetic Patients' Support/Education Group to examine patient-focused resources.
- Patient-held notes.

Reed et al. (2002) discuss their large project which involved a wide range of agencies and included older people, and which developed practice in the area of 'going home from hospital'. The study used three workshops in one English health district, with 71 participants. Group members were also required to carry out some activities between workshops. Workshop 1 discussed the planned research schedule and introduced the basic concepts of AI. Participants were asked the 'miracle question': they were asked to imagine that a miracle had happened overnight and now every hospital discharge went well every time. They were then asked to tell the interviewer:

- What would be different about the world after the miracle?
- What would be in place?
- What would be happening?
- What would the results be?

Notes from the interviews were sent to the coordinators prior to workshop 2, where these interview data were analysed by the group using the nominal group technique. The key themes were the need for understanding, coordination, empowerment and evaluation. A number of provocative propositions were then constructed. These provocative propositions were used at the third workshop when participants were asked to join groups to consider them and their work was developed into action plans. Reed et al. (2002) conclude that while the AI process was useful as a facilitation exercise, the actual project outcomes were difficult to track successfully, as they were working in such as complex, multi-agency setting. As senior management had not participated, it was noted that the 'real' decision makers had not been involved, but the 'networking opportunity' in a positive and blame-free environment was valuable nonetheless.

• • • REFLECTIVE ACTIVITY 1.3 • • •

How might appreciative inquiry help you?

- Think about your own organisation or clinical setting.
- Using the 4-D cycle, think about how you would like things to be.
  - Design: Ask yourself the question 'What do you really want?' from your work.
  - Dream: Dream about how things might improve for you, your patients and clients, your colleagues and the organisation.
  - Design: What would you need to do to make things better? Who would you need to convince? Who would you need to collaborate with? What new networks would you need to establish?
  - Destiny: Once established, how would you evaluate and demonstrate the benefits? What extra work might you need to do to embed and sustain you new practices?

Summary

AR originated as a recognisable entity with Kurt Lewin, who was concerned with developing techniques applicable to the real world for generating change in behaviour (Lewin 1966). Philosophically, AR has been linked to the work of the critical theorists, who sought to change social and economic relations with overtly political action. The long history and methodological diversity of AR is reflected in numerous writers' development of the original concepts and, as Greenwood and Levin (1998) argue, the diffusion of AR ideas is a success story for the movement. While there are many strands, the key point is not which strand you favour as a matter of orthodoxy, but which will work for you in your setting or workplace.

Further reading

These books relate to key issues discussed in the text above, and will be useful as further reading to illustrate the diversity of action research approaches

Coghlan, D and Brannick, T (2010) *Doing action research in your own organisation* (3rd edition). London: Sage.

Cooperrider, D L and Whitney, D (2005) *Appreciative inquiry: A positive revolution in change*. San Francisco, CA: Berrett-Koehler.

Koch, T and Kralik, D (2006) *Participatory action research in healthcare*. Oxford: Blackwell.

Morrow, R A and Brown, D D (1994) *Critical theory and methodology*. London: Sage.
Reed, J (2007) *Appreciative inquiry: Research for change*. London: Sage.
Tyson, L (2006) *Critical theory today* (2nd edition). London: Routledge.

Useful websites

Action Research Resources: www.scu.edu.au/schools/gcm/ar/arhome.html has a number of useful resources.

Actionresearch.net: http://people.bath.ac.uk/edsajw/ has a number of useful links and resources.

Appreciative Inquiry Commons: http://appreciativeinquiry.case.edu/ has a number of useful resources on AI.

Appreciative Inquiry Consulting: www.ai-consulting.co.uk/ has a number of useful resources and video clips on AI.

Centre for Action Research in Professional Practice (CARPP) , University of Bath: www.bath.ac.uk/carpp/.

Collaborative Action Research Network (CARN): www.did.stu.mmu.ac.uk/carnnew/.

Kurt Lewingroups, experiential learning and action research: www.infed.org/thinkers/et-lewin.htm.

New Paradigm Consulting: www.new-paradigm.co.uk/index.htm has a number of useful resources on AI.

Social and Organisational Learning as Action Research, University of the West of England: www.uwe.ac.uk/solar/.

Action research journal websites

Action Research: http://arj.sagepub.com/

Action Research International (online journal): www.scu.edu.au/schools/gcm/ar/ari/arihome.html

Educational Action Research: www.informaworld.com/smpp/title~content=t716100708

References

Argyris, M and Schön, D (1974) *Theory in practice: Increasing professional effectiveness*. San Francisco, CA: Jossey-Bass.

Bronner, S E and Kellner, D K (1989) Introduction. In S E Bronner and D K Kellner (eds), *Critical theory and society: A reader*. London: Routledge, Chapter 1.

Carr, W and Kemmis, S (1986) *Becoming critical: Education, knowledge and action research*. London: The Falmer Press.

Coghlan, D and Brannick, T (2010) *Doing action research in your own organisation* (3rd edition). London: Sage.

Cooperrider, D L (2008) Going green: Maximum velocity through AI's sustainable design factory. Available online at:http://appreciativeinquiry.case.edu/intro/comment.cfm (accessed 6/2/2009).

Cooperrider, D L and Whitney, D (2005) *Appreciative inquiry: A positive revolution in change*. San Francisco, CA: Berrett-Koehler.

Cooperrider, DL, Whitney, D and Stavros, J M (2005) *Appreciative inquiry handbook: The first in a series of AI workbooks for leaders of change*. Brunswick, OH: Crown Custom Publishing.

Dickens, L and Watkins, K (1999) Action research: Rethinking Lewin. *Management Learning* 30(2): 127–140.

Fals Borda, O (2006) Participatory (action) research in social theory: Origins and challenges. In P Reason and H Bradbury (eds) , *Handbook of action research* (2nd edition). London: Sage, Chapter 2.

Greenwood, DJ and Levin, M (1998) *Introduction to action research: Social research for social change*. London: Sage.

Griffiths, M (1994) Autobiography, **feminsim** and the practice of action research. *Educational Action Research* 2(1): 71–83.

Guilar, J and Start, K (2001) Optimizing diabetes care: The appreciative inquiry method. *Practice Nursing* 12(3): 84–85.

Habermas, J (1981/1987) *The theory of communicative action*. London: Beacon Press.

Healy, K (2001) Participatory action research and social work. *International Social Work* 44(1): 93–105.

Heron, J (2001) Transpersonal co-operative inquiry. In P Reason and H Bradbury (eds), *Handbook of action research: Participative inquiry and practice*. London: Sage, Chapter 32.

Heron, J and Reason, P (2006) The practice of co-operative inquiry: Research 'with' rather than 'on' people. In P Reason and H Bradbury (eds), *Handbook of action research* (2nd edition). London: Sage, Chapter 12.

Hollingsworth, S (1997) Killing the angel in academe: Feminist praxis in action research. *Educational Action Research* 5(3): 483–502.

Kellner, D (1989) *Critical theory, Marxism and modernity*. Oxford: Polity Press.

Kemmis, S (1996) Emancipatory aspirations in a postmodern era. In O Zuber-Skerritt (ed.), *New directions in action research*. London: The Falmer Press, Chapter 12.

Kemmis, S (2006) Exploring the relevance of critical theory for action research: Emancipatory action research in the footsteps of Jürgen Habermas. In P Reason and H Bradbury (eds), *Handbook of action research* (2nd edition). London: Sage, Chapter 8.

Kemmis, S and McTaggart, R (eds) (1990) *The action research planner*. Geelong, Vic.: Deakin University Press.

Koch, T and Kralik, D (2006) *Participatory action research in healthcare*. Oxford: Blackwell.

Lather, P (1988) Feminist perspectives on empowering research methodologies. *Women's Studies International Forum* 11(6): 569–581.

Lather, P (1991) *Getting smart: Feminist research and pedagogy with/in the postmodern*. London: Routledge.

Lewin, K (1946) Action research and minority problems. *Journal of Social Issues* 2(4): 34–46.

Lewin, K (1966) Group decisions and social change. In E E Maccoby, T M Newcomb and E L Hartley (eds), *Readings in social psychology*. London: Methuen, (pp. 546–563).

Lewis, J and Van Tiem, D (2004) Appreciative inquiry: A view of a glass half full. *Performance Improvement* 43(8): 19–24.

Maguire, P (2006) Uneven ground: **Feminisms** and action research. In P Reason and H Bradbury (eds), *Handbook of action research* (2nd edition). London: Sage, Chapter 5.

Marcuse, H (1989) Philosophy and critical theory. In S E Bronner and D K Kellner (eds), *Critical theory and society: A reader*. London: Routledge, Chapter 5.

McNiff, J (1988) *Action research: Principles and practice*. London: Routledge.

McNiff, J and Whitehead, J (2002) *Action research: Principles and practice* (2nd edition). London: Routledge.

Meyer, J E (1993) New paradigm research in practice: The trials and tribulations of action research. *Journal of Advanced Nursing* 18: 1066–1072.

Moore, M (2008) Appreciative inquiry: The why? The what? The how? *Practice Development in Health Care* 7(4): 214–220. DOI: 10.1002/pdh.270.

Morrow, R A and Brown, D D (1994) *Critical theory and methodology* (3rd edition). London: Sage.

Oakley, A (1981) Interviewing women: A contradiction in terms. In H Roberts (ed.), *Doing feminist research*. London: Routledge and Kegan Paul, Chapter 2.

Oliver, C (2005) Critical appreciative inquiry as intervention in organisational discourse. In E Peck (ed.), *Organisational development in healthcare: Approaches, innovations, achievements*. Oxford: Radcliffe, Chapter 12.

Piran, N (2001) Reinhabiting the body. ***Feminism** and Psychology* 11(2): 172–176.

Reason, P (ed.) (1994a) *Participation in human inquiry*. London: Sage.

Reason, P (1994b) Three approaches to participative inquiry. In N K Denzin and Y S Lincoln (eds), *Handbook of qualitative research*. Thousand Oaks, CA: Sage, Chapter 20.

Reason, P and Bradbury, H (eds) (2006) *Handbook of action research* (2nd edition). London: Sage.

Reed, J, Pearson, P, Douglas, B, Swinburne, S and Wilding, H (2002) Going home from hospital: An appreciative inquiry study. *Health and Social Care in the Community* 10(1): 36–45.

Seel, R (2008) Introduction to appreciative inquiry. Available online at: http://www.new-paradigm.co.uk/introduction_to_ai.htm (accessed 6/2/2009).

Sitzia, J (2001) Barriers to research utilization: The clinical setting and nurses themselves. *European Journal of Oncology Nursing* 5(3): 154–164.

Stringer, E (1999) *Action research: A handbook for practitioners* (2nd edition). Thousand Oaks, CA: Sage.

Torbert, WR (2006) The practice of action inquiry. In P Reason and H Bradbury (eds), *Handbook of action research* (2nd edition). London: Sage, Chapter 18.

Waterman, H, Tillen, D, Dickson, R and de Koning, K (2001): Action research: a systematic review and guidance for assessment. *Health Technology Assessment*. 5(23)

Webb, C (1993) Feminist research: Definitions, methodology/methods and evaluation. *Journal of Advanced Nursing* 18: 416–423.

Weiner, G (2004) Critical action research and third wave feminism: A meeting of paradigms. *Educational Action Research* 12(4): 631–644.

Winter, R and Munn-Giddings, C (2001) *A handbook for action research in health and social care*. London: Routledge.

2

DISCUSSION, DEBATE AND CONTROVERSY SURROUNDING ACTION RESEARCH

Graham R Williamson

Chapter objectives

There is much controversy surrounding action research. It is open to criticism as 'not scientific', not objective and open to bias due to the proximity of researchers and participants. However, a contrary argument views action research as a 'new **paradigm**' approach, a different worldview of research, which therefore does not need to subscribe to its critics' demand for rigour as in traditional research approaches. This chapter will explore these issues, framed in the debates concerning:

- qualitative and quantitative research and the mixed methods debate;
- scientific research standards and action research;
- validity, generalisability, credibility and **reflexivity**;
- evaluation studies, audit and AR;
- critical voices in healthcare action research.

Introduction

It is characteristic of research methods textbooks that they rehearse arguments about the different research **paradigms**, these being quantitative and qualitative research. For convenience, they are generally portrayed as opposite, even opposing ways of viewing the world for research purposes, and although in reality the issues are not as straightforward as that, this is still a common way of presenting the two **paradigms**. However, as we shall see, contemporary thinking has come to emphasise the potential synergies that exist rather than the conflicts.

Research paradigms and the mixed methods debate

Quantitative research is concerned with measurement of external phenomena, using hypotheses to manipulate or analyse variables, with structured instruments to collect data such as questionnaires or rating scales. Numerical information is collected which can be analysed statistically. Although there is controversy and debate about this, Hammersley (1995) notes that quantitative research is frequently associated with **positivism**, a school of thought based on the traditions of the **natural sciences**, which takes the 'scientific method' of observation and testing and the verifiability principle as the only claims to knowledge; that is, that only logical, mathematical understanding and statements that have empirical proof are acceptable as evidence.

This **positivism** was applied to social science research from its background in the **natural sciences** in the late nineteenth century by August Comte, and its influence continued into the twentieth century. A school known as the Vienna Circle held influence until the 1950s, when critical voices began to examine social science research differently. Important figures in twentieth-century **positivism** were Hahn, Schlick and Wittgenstein, whose concerns were broadly to argue against abstract thinking and to focus more on a concern with 'reality'. Critics included Popper, who argued that falsification rather than verifiability was important (that is, that we can accept some statements not only if we can prove them, but also if we cannot disprove them) and Ayer. From the 1960s, the **positivistic** assumptions of being able to discover objective facts about the world faded as guiding principles in the social sciences. A key part in the demise of **positivism** was Kuhn's) work, *The Structure of Scientific Revolutions* (2nd edition, 1970), in which he argued that far from being about discovery of objective facts, **natural sciences** progressed not by the gradual accumulation of knowledge, but by great leaps in understanding as a result of challenges to the accepted ways of doing things (Hammersley 1995). Common examples of quantitative research in the healthcare field are randomised controlled trials and large-scale surveys.

In contrast to this **positivist** approach is the qualitative **paradigm**, which emphasises not the objectivity and deduction of a quantitative approach, but explores meaning and constructing understanding with participants in their own, 'real' worlds (Parahoo 2006). This takes an inductive approach and generally collects data using interviews to produce text that can be transcribed and analysed for themes. Various schools of qualitative research have emerged in the twentieth century, for example phenomenology, grounded theory, ethnography and feminist research, all of which take their starting point not in trying to test a **hypothesis** but instead in gaining an in-depth understanding of some aspect of the culture, beliefs and behaviour of participants. They are part of a qualitative, **interpretivist** or constructionist **paradigm** which emphasises how humans construct their own interpretations of life.

At the heart of the differences between **paradigms** lie questions of ontology and epistemology. Epistemology asks the question 'How is it possible to gain knowledge of the world?' whereas ontology asks 'What kinds of things exist in the world?' (Hughes and Sharrock 1997). Ontologically speaking, a quantitative approach would lead us to the answer 'What exists is what can be proven' whereas a qualitative approach might leads us to a more relative answer that this would depend on who you asked, at what time and under what circumstances. The epistemological concerns of each **paradigm** would also be different as a quantitative approach would use the testing of hypotheses and a qualitative approach would look to interpret and understand the experiences of individuals and groups. The methods of data collection by which evidence is gained will also differ in line with the philosophical **paradigm** used in a research study, and how these link to the **paradigm** is known as the methodology. For example, in a randomised controlled trial evaluating a new medication for treating high blood pressure, a large number of participants would have their blood pressure measured over periods of time, and the measurements of those taking the new treatment might be compared with those taking a placebo (an inert compound in a similar tablet form). The measurements would allow statistical comparisons to be made between the groups in order to prove the **hypothesis** that the new treatment was more effective than a placebo. Thus the method of data collection would be quantitative: by how much did the mean blood pressure differ between the groups and could this be shown to be a statistically significant difference? In a qualitative study, where the interest was in patients' experiences of having high blood pressure, the focus would be to understand the meaning of the illness for sufferers. Data might be collected in individual or group interviews, using tape recordings of conversations. These interviews would be transcribed and analysed for themes. The data collection method is thus wholly qualitative as there are no numbers involved and the purpose is different: not to test a **hypothesis** but to find out and understand more about the experiences of those interviewed.

Although researchers *may* choose to use qualitative or quantitative research because of a deep-seated personal preference or a political bias, actually the research question or objective drives the choice of research **paradigm** and subsequent methods. Instead where the focus of the research question/objective is change, an action research study might be constructed that involved participants in their own care and treatment, by, for example, their choosing a diet and exercise regime in combination with medication to lower their blood pressure.

Mixing methods and triangulation

Latterly, the above **paradigm** distinctions have been relaxed by some researchers seeking to look beyond what has been characterised as a situation of conflict between qualitative and quantitative researchers, where quantitative research was characterised as measurement-obsessed and irrelevant for exploring meaning, and qualitative research was described as 'touchy-feely', biased, subjective and lacking generalisability. In fact, it seems as if a consensus now exists that the differences are exaggerated, and that there are gains to be made from incorporating the two perspectives in studies (Parahoo 2006): the strengths of each can be used synergistically, while acknowledging 'weaknesses'. Arguably, complex phenomena require more complex approaches than can be achieved by single-methods studies, and so combining methods in mixed-methods studies is now acceptable in a way which may not have been possible several years ago.

The concept of triangulation can be applied to mixing methods, just as it can be applied to using two or more methods from the same **paradigm**. While the original meaning of the term 'triangulation' comes from trigonometry as a way of measuring the location of one point from two others, it is useful as it indicates how various methods in social science research can be used to gain depth in the understanding of complex phenomena (Williamson 2005) and increase the credibility the findings. Denzin (1989) outlines four methods of triangulation. These are:

- data triangulation, involving many different data collection sources;
- investigator triangulation, involving more than one researcher to collect and analyse data;
- theoretical triangulation, involving more than one theoretical approach (for example, Marxist, feminist and/or phenomenological perspectives) to interpret findings;
- methodological triangulation, of which there are two different types. 'Within-method' triangulation involves using different data collection methods within one **paradigm.** 'Between-method' triangulation involves the use of qualitative and quantitative data collection approaches within one study to investigate the same phenomenon.

In Williamson (2005), I drew on Denzin's (1989) work to discuss triangulation as offering the potential to overcome the inadequacies of each **paradigm**, although researchers should not expect *identical* findings to emerge from different data collection methods, which would be impossible when the perspectives and theoretical assumptions behind the methods differ. Instead, methodological triangulation allows a wider or more complete picture to emerge than that presented by single-methods work – issues may emerge from one data collection method that were not in evidence in another. For example, consider again the study above of a new blood pressure treatment. Testing the blood pressure reduction of a new treatment compared to another treatment or a placebo will not tell us what it is like for patients to take it. For that, interviews with patients would be required. Combining the two methods (quantitative testing and qualitative interpretation) would give a more complete picture of whether the new treatment works and whether patients will actually be able to tolerate it.

Mixing methods in action research

Box 2.1

Research example

In Williamson (2005), I outlined how I used a range of methods in an action research study, and how using the different methods challenged me to think more carefully and thoroughly about the findings I attained from the participants. I was developing the role of lecturer-practitioners in nursing (LPs – a work role common in nursing where the post-holder works in clinical practice as well as in a lecturing role in the local university teaching students) (Williamson et al. 2004). These roles are described in the literature as being difficult and stressful (Williamson 2004), and as well as introducing supportive activities, I was interested in uncovering new knowledge about occupational stress and burnout. Participants in focus groups discussed how stressed they were, but using quantitative measures of occupational stress and burnout indicated that the LPs were no worse off than national averages, and there was a clear dichotomy in data from the two **paradigms**. Obviously, if I had only taken data from either **paradigm,** I would have reported findings that did not fully examine the reality of occupational stress and burnout for these workers. Interpretations and recommendations may therefore not have been fully representative as a result. The methods used were complementary rather than antagonistic. Neither method was 'better' than the other or produced 'superior' findings and one did not prove or disprove the other. Using triangulation enabled the conclusion that LPs found aspects of their work stressful and potentially a source of burnout, but they considered themselves to be survivors who were largely thriving as a group.

In practice, any data collection method can be used in action research studies, and although it would be very unusual to see action research using wholly quantitative measures, it is theoretically possible. However, as it relies on a participatory and **democratic** relationship between researcher and participants, action research fits more 'securely' into the qualitative, interpretive or constructivist **paradigm**. For Koch and Kralik (2006), it is about inclusiveness in the construction of knowledge that leads to action, and it is this latter element, the requirement to take action, that has led to its categorisation as a **paradigm** in itself – a third **paradigm**.

A third paradigm?

As noted in Chapter 1, Reason (1988) uses the term 'new **paradigm** research' to illustrate how AR differs from traditional forms of inquiry, requiring participation and collaboration and a changed worldview (Reason 1994a). New **paradigm** research is thus critical of other research traditions that find problems but no solutions, and stands outside the 'quantitative versus qualitative' debate by acting to address perceived problems by those closest to them. Traditional research approaches are inadequate, as they produce abstract rather than practical thinking: they do not (directly) change anything and produce only academic papers (Heron and Reason 2006). It can be argued that both qualitative and quantitative researchers are 'outsiders' to the context of the research. A quantitative researcher, conducting the above drug trial example for anti-hypertensive medication, would stand outside the 'reality' of having high blood pressure. It would not be necessary or desirable to experience **hypertension** in order to collect data about it. Although that researcher may have made a career of such studies, the need for objectivity should mean that data are accurately collected and analysed, and results and conclusions interpreted accordingly. A qualitative researcher seeking to understand the meaning or experience of **hypertension** would similarly be collecting data, and although their perspective would be from much closer to the participants, they would still be collecting data and disappearing from the participants' reality to analyse it. While feminist researchers, for example, may argue that their standpoint as women makes them very close to their participants, closer than others, arguably they are still frequently academic researchers collecting data. Action research is different from qualitative and quantitative research because the researcher becomes an equal participant in groups with others, with those caring for and users diagnosed with **hypertension**, and it is the collective understanding thus generated that also indicates the courses of action to be taken.

While it is the case that much action research is conducted by external researchers who become insiders to a large extent, it is also the case that many action researchers are insiders to start with, attempting beneficial change for themselves and others who share some social concern (see Chapter 4). As Reason (1988: 1) puts it, 'Who was that research I saw you with last night? That was no research, that was my life!' So, action research can be described as a third **paradigm** because of the involvement of researchers and their collaboration with participants, and their explicit remit of changing for the better aspects of the clinical and/or social worlds of participants.

Of course, these issues are not without controversy, and some of these controversies are explored below.

Validity in action research

AR does not use the accepted principles of the scientific method, such as reliability (it is replicable by others), **validity** (it describes a 'true' state of affairs and/or is generalisable to other settings) and generalisability (research findings are applicable to a wide variety of contexts) to generate law-like theories of nature, and it does not require the separation of the researcher from the 'field'. Instead it requires the researcher to work in participation with others, and action researchers are clear that this involvement is essential for changing social reality/clinical practice. Critics might argue that this means that action researchers produce accounts that are 'coloured' by their proximity to the research, and cannot separate their involvement from the reality of the project. This is an important criticism that can apply to the internal **validity** of data collection methods, which must be acknowledged and addressed. However, Waterman et al. (2001) argue that this intimacy is essential in mediating change in the situation. Titchen (1995) notes that all qualitative researchers are open to these claims, but that it is the personal perception of reality that is important. According to Titchen: 'All actors must use their biases, beliefs and values in their action. If they did not, they would be unable to act' (Titchen 1995: 40). Indeed, personal interpretations, through reflection, narrative and **reflexivity** (see below), frequently provide legitimate background motivations for action researchers involved in changing practice.

Morton-Cooper (2000) believes that it is of little value in AR to search for absolute reliability, as it is too 'subjective' a process. However, what is important is that the work has 'cultural validity' (2000: 85), that is, it is recognisable by the practitioners as broadly appropriate if the findings 'make sense' to readers. In this respect, AR is about illustrating problems at the 'sharp end' of practice, as well as generating ideas about how other practitioners can address their own problems in their own settings.

For Waterman (1995), traditional 'scientific' standards of judgement are inappropriate for AR. Instead, action researchers should discuss **reflexivity** in the data collection and analysis of their studies, and 'bring the situation to life' (1995: 22) so that the context can be fully appreciated by readers. Koch and Harrington (1998) go further, arguing that it is inappropriate to import quantitative concepts like reliability and **validity** into qualitative research (in which

paradigm they include action research). However, Reason (1994b) argues that 'validity' is an important concept for AR, but in need of reinterpretation for action researchers because it rests on the collaborative encounter with experience. Assessing **validity** depends on the researcher's 'critical subjectivity': their high-quality, critical and self-aware judgements. This involves action researchers accepting their knowledge of the situation as a subjective experience rather than trying to suppress it, and articulating this awareness by attending to the ground on which they are standing. There will be many different versions of 'reality' but this diversity can be overcome by frequently cycling and recycling between action and reflection so that issues are examined in different ways, exploring the authenticity of participation within the group, using self-development techniques and establishing norms, and enabling the group to challenge the action researcher facilitator and one another's interpretations.

Multiple cycling is supported by Waterman (1998), who describes this as one of the prime indicators of 'validity' in action research. Although critical of applying concepts from 'scientific' research to AR, she uses the term 'validity' as a 'yardstick' to assess the extent to which AR studies have:

- **dialectical validity** (concerned with changing practice, and the movement between different stages in the spiral framework);
- critical **validity** (concerned with moral responsibilities); and
- reflexive **validity** (concerned with recognising and valuing the influence of oneself in the research process).

These aspects of 'validity' in AR are not uncomplicated, however, and continually generate uncertainties and contradictions. Titchen (1995) discusses three other methods of ensuring the **validity** of AR. These are, first, methodological triangulation, where data are collected from different sources. When findings from different data sources agree, the researcher can be confident in their consistency and completeness (Cutcliffe and McKenna 1999), and there will be a wider and deeper perspective in the researchers' interpretation (Denzin 1989). Second, wherever possible there should be prolonged and persistent observation in the field, so that those reading AR accounts can be sure that the researcher has a prolonged period of collaboration with participants. Third, although participants should be fully involved in developing understanding in the study, where a researcher writes an account, participant verification should take place, and participants should be asked to check the data and findings for accuracy and completeness. Morton-Cooper (2000) goes further, saying that verification should also be by outsiders: significant disinterested colleagues should be involved to see if they agree or disagree with the findings from the various data sets. Producing valid research reports in AR is thus a highly collaborative exercise (see Chapter 8).

McNiff et al. (1996) have some practical points concerning procedures for ensuring **validity** in AR. In writing up the project, they argue, the researcher should be able to demonstrate that they have developed new meaning and new understanding by working collaboratively with other participants. The AR account should also be able to show how participants' tacit knowledge has been made explicit. As the project has been about enabling participants to do this in order to change or develop some aspect of practice, the researcher should be able to discuss this and in doing so acknowledge their accountability to participants. Waterman (1998) discusses this as a moral responsibility, and extends this responsibility to patients and clients, arguing that staff have a duty to improve services. However, she also argues that in action research it is inappropriate to judge the **validity** of the project solely by the extent to which change is implemented, as excessive volumes of change may overload and unsettle staff.

Interpreting action research outside its own context

Although not the only important element in AR, the application to other settings is a central element in practice development (Waterman et al. 2001). AR work cannot be generalised in the **positivist** research sense, but it is likely that the work can be interpreted in similar situations in other organisations, and so can be relevant elsewhere. Similarly, social science research does not produce findings with the kind of predictive power of the **natural sciences**, but it does produce medium-range findings which are generally or reasonably close enough to the position in other situations and settings to allow for broad generalisation (Williams 2000). In that sense it can be transferable rather than generalisable to other contexts.

Credibility in action research: acknowledging or suppressing the impact of proximity?

Titchen (1995) notes that AR requires a high level of self-awareness and skill so that personal 'biases' are switched off in order to accurately record and evaluate practical changes in a theoretical account. She advocates that the researcher be continually personally challenging, asking: 'Was I really doing that?' (1995: 41), recognising their ethical obligation as researchers to be self-aware and acknowledge their impact on others. However, the AR literature on this issue of how proximity to the research might impact on the account produced shows an apparent conflict between switching off personal biases and acknowledging them (Koch and Harrington 1998). Bradbury and Reason (2006) argue that action researchers should acknowledge their subjectivity, and that a more useful term to describe this self-validation is 'credibility': the researcher must acknowledge that AR involves **reflexivity**, and be able to produce an account which is not just their own perception of events.

Credibility is the extent to which processes were followed which allow the reader to trust the account. Greenwood and Levin (1998) identify two kinds of credible knowledge: internal and external. Internal credibility is fundamentally important as it demonstrates that the AR account is credible to those who collaborated in the project. The connection to the local situation is clear, as should be the extent of change. External credibility concerns how far others are convinced by the account. This is more complex, as the challenge to AR, from an unenlightened reader, is that the proximity of the researcher can be dismissed as offering a 'biased' account (see also Chapter 8).

Greenwood and Levin (1998) argue that there are three principles required for credible AR:

- 'Workability' means that actions taken in the research solve a real-world problem.
- These tangible results can be interpreted and constructed to offer meaning and understanding of what has occurred.
- The accounts produced have transcontextual meaning: that is, they have relevance to people in other areas, not in an abstract sense, but when the contexts of reader and writer are taken into account.

••• REFLECTIVE ACTIVITY 2.1 •••

Consider ways in which you would justify using action research to (a) a sceptical colleague, and (b) a 'traditional' researcher. Drawing on the discussion above, write yourself some notes for both 'audiences'.

Reflexivity in action research

Reflexivity is important in all qualitative research, but is especially so in action research. It is a continuous process undertaken by the researcher of reflecting on their actions and behaviour in relation to participants and the research process. The interplay of individuals in groups, with organisations or in the community, with participants who have differing views, backgrounds and aspirations is complex and requires acknowledgement as it affects the interpretation and understanding of events in the research study (Parahoo 2006). This is a difficult process, and arguably requires a great deal of thought and effort, including the use of a reflective diary and time in which to explore and examine these aspects of collaborative working. As it is certain that a two-way process of influencing the research context will take place between participants, an understanding of the impact of this process by the writer of accounts, whether for academic or publication purposes is essential. '**Reflexivity**' is the term given to making this explicit. It is described as giving accounts of action research studies to add credibility (Parahoo 2006).

Evaluation studies, audit and action research

Evaluation studies (process and **outcome evaluations**) are designed to discover whether some particular activity or service is meeting the needs of clients and staff, and meeting the aims and objectives specified in advance. Audit has a similar focus. Both must collect data (from qualitative and/or quantitative perspectives) and both are aimed at a particular situation or practice, but while audit has become a routine activity imbedded in many aspects of healthcare provision, evaluation can often be more *adhoc*, although the importance of both is growing with the need for evidence for practice and clinical governance (Parahoo 2006). Audits frequently record whether a change has taken place, but evaluation seeks to discover why, as well as what, has changed.

There are many different means of conducting evaluation research and audit (Moule and Goodman 2009), but while there are similarities between these methods and action research, such as the focus on change, the collection of data in a systematic process, the focus on a particular situation and the views of those in the situation, there are also key differences. Audit and evaluation tend to be more managerial tools than the attempt at empowerment and **emancipation** inherent in many AR studies. There is no attempt in audit and evaluation to foster genuine collaboration and an equal dialogue between participants and researchers. Participants are not involved in all stages of the process in audit or evaluation: they do not set the agenda or direction for change, or play a part in the production of knowledge as they would do in AR. The task focus of audit and evaluation can militate against the abstract theorising and consciousness-raising that can take place in AR (Koch and Kralik 2006).

A further level of distinction is provided by the NHS Research Ethics Service (2008), which has some interesting distinctions between research, audit and service evaluation. These are outlined in Table 2.1.

Although it is useful for those needing to decide whether to submit their work for ethical clearance, Table 2.1 simplifies these approaches and this may

Table 2.1 Definitions of research, audit and service evaluation (adapted from NHS Research Ethics Service 2008)

Research	Audit	Service evaluation
Attempts to derive generalisable new knowledge, including to generating and testing hypotheses.	Designed and conducted to produce information to inform delivery of best care.	Designed and conducted solely to define or judge current care.
Quantitative research – designed to test a hypothesis. Qualitative research – identifies/explores themes following established methodology.	Designed to find out if a service reaches a predetermined standard.	Designed to find out the standard a service achieves.
Addresses clearly defined questions, aims and objectives.	Measures against a standard.	Measures current service without reference to a standard.
Quantitative research – may involve evaluating or comparing interventions, particularly new ones. Qualitative research – usually involves studying how interventions and relationships are experienced.	Involves an intervention already in use.	Involves an intervention already in use.
Usually involves collecting data that are additional to those for routine care.	Usually involves analysis of existing data, but may include administration of simple interview or questionnaire.	Usually involves analysis of existing data, but may include administration of simple interview or questionnaire.
Quantitative research – study design may involve allocating patients to intervention groups. Qualitative research uses a clearly defined sampling framework underpinned by conceptual or theoretical justifications.	No allocation to intervention groups.	No allocation to intervention groups.
May involve randomisation.	No randomisation.	No randomisation.

not be completely helpful for researchers designing studies. A key issue that relates to the differences between audit, evaluation and AR is the intent of the study. Where the primary aim of research is to derive new knowledge, audit and service evaluation measure or investigate levels of care. Research is to find out what we should be doing; audit is to find out what we are doing (NHS Research Ethics Service 2008). Thus AR is clearly a research technique because of its focus on generating new knowledge *and* using an established methodology with an underpinning theoretical justification (albeit that, in view of the aforementioned controversies, changing practice is not mentioned by NHS Research Ethics Service 2008), whereas audit and evaluation are 'other' functions of healthcare inquiry.

Critical voices in action research

Throughout discussions of action research methodologies and approaches there is often an implicit belief that the project will achieve beneficial outcomes for those concerned, and that in acting to facilitate change, action researchers are facilitating a group process that is essentially benign. This may not be the case. What happens if participants actually don't want the empowerment and **emancipation** that researchers may think they need? Despite attempts to ensure otherwise, action researchers can be, or can be perceived to be, in a position of significantly more power than the participants in their studies. Criticism of action research can be made at several levels. Three key areas of concern for action researchers to bear in mind are:

- interpersonal conflict;
- organisational conflicts;
- political disagreements.

••• REFLECTIVE ACTIVITY 2.2 •••

Before reading the following discussion of these potential areas of conflict, think about your ideas for an AR project and its context. Think about the participants you want to join you and the organisational structure in which you will be working. Can you identify sources of conflict that are:

- Interpersonal?
- Organisational?
- Political?

Make some notes on them. What strategies will you employ to avoid, minimise, or work around these factors in order to improve your chances of success?

At the interpersonal level, there may be conflicts within groups and between group members about what are the best ways to proceed. This is likely to happen in most studies and, if occurring at a low level, can be managed by good facilitation and working towards consensus (see Chapter 6). Koch and Kralik (2006) argue that conflict is not always negative and can in fact be a means by which groups progress and develop their ideas and strategies. If conflicts cannot be resolved, then at least they should be discussed openly and participants can 'agree to differ'. It will be beneficial in clarifying at the outset what are the participants' expectations of taking part, what they hope to gain and what their personal agendas are. These can be agreed as, for example, a set of ground rules early on in the study.

Organisational conflicts may take many forms, but essentially the action research groups may experience difficulties in trying to change practice and may come into conflict with existing power relations. Participants are much more exposed to potential harm from this than those in other types of study as it is usually much easier to identify group members than in other types of study. The micro-political organisational climate and culture are very important and researchers and participants must be sensitive to these aspects of organisational life to avoid negative personal and career consequences for themselves, which may be wide-reaching and serious (Coghlan and Brannick 2010; Williamson and Prosser 2002).

Arguably, the organisational culture prevalent in the NHS, with its emphasis on improving quality while reducing costs, means that AR may be another means for managers to ensure that workers are compliant with managerial priorities. Reflective practice may be used as a method for individualising and controlling the workforce to ensure that managerial goals are internalised (Hart 1996). Hart (1996) is pessimistic that AR in such a hierarchical culture can be genuinely **democratic**, but argues that it has potential if used appropriately to empower a largely female workforce. Elsewhere (Hart and Bond 1995), argue that 'new **paradigm**' research has emancipatory and empowering potential for nurses, based on its critical perspective, but if used wrongly, it can be subverted and used to exercise more subtle forms of power over already 'powerless' nursing staff.

As well as micro-political or small 'p' political, disagreements within organisations, there may also be ideological disagreements about political issues, or large 'P' politics. Koch and Kralik (2006) discuss this in the context of their work, particularly when facilitating feminist participatory research, where they found that, in the short term, their participants were actually disempowered and disorganised, as the study undermined coping strategies that had allowed their female participants to cope with years of gender-based violence. They conclude that the complexities and challenges of others' lives must be taken into account in AR, and to impose feminist ideology would have been inappropriate for their study at that stage. It must always be remembered that just because participants share the same space and want change, they do not necessarily believe everything that the researcher does, and may even disagree fundamentally with one's political perspective. Care must be taken to establish how far participants want to go, and consent must be continually negotiated so that the direction of the research is always clear to participants (Williamson and Prosser 2002) (this is explored further in Chapter 7).

Summary

Action research can be characterised as a third **paradigm**, outside the traditional arguments concerning qualitative and quantitative research, because AR is about generating new knowledge as well as changing practice. It is also distinct from audit and evaluation studies, which are seen as increasingly important for healthcare evidence. Changing practice is a particular goal in healthcare settings, as is uncovering new knowledge. AR is not without the potential for interpersonal, organisational and political conflicts, which can have a significant impact on studies. Consequently, action researchers need to both plan for and manage them. If consensus is established, AR can be powerful and effective in securing collaboration and changing practice.

Further reading

Coghlan, D and Brannick, T (2010) *Doing action research in your own organisation* (3rd edition). London: Sage. An excellent discussion of the key issues as suggested by the title.

Hammersley, M (1995) *The politics of social research*. London: Sage. A key text exploring political issues in research.

Hughes, J A and Sharrock, W W (1997) *The philosophy of social research* (3rd edition). London: Longman Pearson. A key text exploring the philosophical distinctions between qualitative and quantitative research.

Jupp, V (ed.) (2006) *The SAGE dictionary of social research methods*. London: Sage. Very good on a range of approaches to research.

Parahoo, K (2006) *Nursing research, principles and process issues* (2nd edition). Basingstoke: Palgrave Macmillan. A good introductory nursing research textbook although limited on action research.

Waterman, H, Marshall, M, Noble, J, Davies, H, Walshe, K, Sheaff, R and Elwyn, G (2007) The role of action research in the investigation and diffusion of innovations in health care: The PRIDE project. Qualitative Health Research 17(3): 373–381. DOI: 10.1177/1049732306298976. Discussion and analysis of strengths and weaknesses of action research in relation to the investigation and practical implementation of innovations in healthcare.

Williamson, G R (2005) Illustrating triangulation in mixed-methods nursing research. *Nurse Researcher* 12(4): 7–18. Discusses the concept of triangulation in data collection and analysis in mixed-methods research and reflects on how this contributes to a deeper understanding.

Williamson, G R, Jenkinson, T and Proctor-Childs, T (2010) *Contexts of contemporary nursing* (2nd edition). Exeter: Leaning Matters. Chapter 8 on evidence-based practice has good introductory material on research concepts and designs for novice researchers.

Williamson, G R and Prosser, S (2002) Action research: Politics, ethics and participation. *Journal of Advanced Nursing* 40(5): 587–593. Explores how organisational politics alters the ethical dimensions of action research. Some strategies are suggested.

Useful websites

Using Google to search for research terms produces millions of hits! In general, sites from recognised US and UK universities will be reasonably trustworthy. Avoid citing Wikepedia in academic work as, although the information may be correct, there are no guarantees because pages can be changed by any registered users at any time!

An Introduction to Qualitative Research by B Hancock (2002): www.trentrdsu.org.uk/cms/uploads/Qualitative%20Research.pdf. A useful short introduction using healthcare examples.

Kipworld:www.kipworld.net. An interesting site by Dr Kip Jones of the Centre for Qualitative Research, Bournemouth University. It explores the links between the creative arts and social science research (performative social science and narrative research).

Research Methods Knowledge Base: www.socialresearchmethods.net/kb/index.php. A web-based text aimed at undergraduate level. Mostly covers quantitative topics but includes a small amount on qualitative issues.

Sage Research Methods online http://srmo.sagepub.com/publicstart;sessionid=5749COE9FB2EA38480E3D6E7E982032?authRejection=true This is an excellent resource with a wealth of information about research methods.

References

Bradbury, H and Reason, P (2006) Broadening the bandwidth of validity: Issues and choice-points for improving the quality of action research. In P Reason and H Bradbury (eds), *Handbook of action research* (2nd edition). London: Sage, Chapter 33.

Coghlan, D and Brannick, T (2010) *Doing action research in your own organisation* (3rd edition). London: Sage.

Cutcliffe, J R and McKenna, H P (1999) Establishing the credibility of qualitative research findings: The plot thickens. *Journal of Advanced Nursing* 30(2): 374–380.

Denzin, N K (1989) *The research act* (3rd edition). London: PrenticeHall.

Greenwood, DJ and Levin, M (1998) *Introduction to action research: Social research for social change*. London: Sage.

Hammersley, M (1995) *The politics of social research*. London: Sage.

Hart, E (1996) Action research as a professionalising strategy: Issues and dilemmas. *Journal of Advanced Nursing* 23(3): 454–461.

Hart, E and Bond, M (1995) Developing action research in nursing. *Nurse Researcher* 2(3): 4–14.

Heron, J and Reason, P (2006) The practice of co-operative inquiry: Research 'with' rather than 'on' people. In P Reason and H Bradbury (eds), *Handbook of action research* (2nd edition). London: Sage, Chapter 12.

Hughes, J A and Sharrock, W W (1997) *The philosophy of social research* (3rd edition). London: Longman Pearson.

Koch, T and Harrington, A (1998) Reconceptualizing rigour: The case for **reflexivity**. *Journal of Advanced Nursing* 28(4): 882–890.

Koch, T and Kralik, D (2006) *Participatory action research in healthcare*. Oxford: Blackwell.

Kuhn, T S (1970) *The structure of scientific revolutions* (2nd edition). Chicago, IL: University of Chicago Press.

McNiff, J, Lomax, P and Whitehead, J (1996) *You and your action research project.* London: Hyde Publications.

Morton-Cooper, A (2000) *Action research in health care.* London: Blackwell Science.

Moule, P and Goodman, M (2009) *Nursing research: An introduction.* London: Sage.

NHS Research Ethics Service (2008) *Defining research.* London: National Patient Safety Agency.

Parahoo, K (2006) *Nursing research, principles and process issues*(2nd edition). Basingstoke: Palgrave Macmillan.

Reason, P (1988) *Human inquiry in action: Developments in new paradigm research.* London: Sage.

Reason, P (ed.) (1994a) *Participation in human inquiry.* London: Sage.

Reason, P (1994b) Three approaches to participative inquiry. In N K Denzin and Y S Lincoln (eds) *Handbook of qualitative research.* Thousand Oaks, CA: Sage, Chapter 20.

Titchen, A (1995) Issues of validity in action research. *Nurse Researcher* 2(3): 38–48.

Waterman, H (1995): Distinguishing between 'traditional' and action research. *Nurse Researcher* 2(3): 15–23.

Waterman, H (1998) Embracing ambiguities and valuing ourselves: Issues of validity in action research. *Journal of Advanced Nursing* 28(1): 101–105.

Williams, M (2000) *Science and social science: An introduction.* London: Routledge.

Williamson, G R (2004) Lecturer practitioners in UK nursing and midwifery: What is the evidence? A systematic review of the literature. *Journal of Clinical Nursing* 13: 787–795.

Williamson, G R (2005) Illustrating triangulation in mixed-methods nursing research. *Nurse Researcher* 12(4): 7–18.

Williamson, G R and Prosser, S (2002) Action research: Politics, ethics and participation. *Journal of Advanced Nursing* 40(5): 587–593.

Williamson, G R, Webb, C and Abelson-Mitchell, N (2004) Developing lecturer-practitioner roles using action research. *Journal of Advanced Nursing* 47(2): 153–164.

SECTION 2

WHY CHOOSE ACTION RESEARCH?

3

ACTION RESEARCH, NURSING AND HEALTHCARE

Graham R Williamson

Chapter objectives

This chapter will explore some of the underpinning ideas concerning the application of action research to nursing and healthcare practice, so in this chapter we will cover theoretical material and research examples from areas including:

- changing practice using action research;
- generating new theory about practice using action research;
- interpersonal relationships in nursing action research;
- participatory action research in healthcare and nursing research – improving 'quality of life' for individuals and communities.

Introduction

Action research is being used in many settings from industry to the developing world. The principles of action research can be identified from projects conducted in these different settings but the culture of bureaucratic healthcare organisations and the context in which people work requires further consideration. One key reason for this is the high degree of autonomy more often enjoyed by other workers compared to those in healthcare, who are constrained by the multidisciplinary nature and organisational features of healthcare settings. This may result in relatively small change projects impacting on other powerful actors (Greenwood 1994), such as, for example, if one healthcare professional group decided to change practice unilaterally that would have impacts on other groups within the NHS. Even so, AR is becoming more widely recognised as a sustainable force for change among diverse communities in global healthcare settings. It is multifaceted, having interpersonal as well as organisational dimensions.

Changing nursing practice using action research

As Bridges and Meyer (2007) argue, action research can be highly effective as a tool for achieving organisational change in healthcare organisations, as a result of its inherent characteristics, which overlap with those of the literature on organisational change. However, this is dependent on engaging managers as well as practitioners in change strategies. Arguably, AR is much more than a tool. It is a philosophical approach to change (see Chapter 1). Identifying it as a tool does not do it full justice but it may be useful to do so in a managerial context. While there is a government rhetoric concerning democratisation of decision making, there still exists a strong command-and-control ethos within the NHS, meaning that the impetus for service change may still come from outside the healthcare professions (Bridges and Meyer 2007). However, as the examples below illustrate, there is still much potential for practitioner-driven change in clinical services, and action research provides a means for facilitating that change.

Hart (1996) notes that a spiral or cyclical AR method is attractive for nurses because it mirrors the nursing process, quality circles, and reflective practice models. Elsewhere, Hart and Bond (1995a) discuss a framework for action research with six elements (see Figure 3.1): reflect on a theme, plan action, take action to change practice, observe and evaluate, reflect, plan (and so on). This schema is primarily intended to facilitate the implementation of change. Once again, similar to Chapter 1, an evaluation of Figure 3.1 indicates that while it gives a structure for planning a study, it is not able to represent fully the spiral, developmental nature of an AR study. Also Hart and Bond (1995a) have moved from a three- or four-stage strategy, as we saw in Chapter 1, to a six-stage one.

Healthcare practitioners disillusioned by the failure of research to provide solutions to workplace problems use AR as 'the over-arching aim of action research has been to improve professional practice and raise standards of service provision' (Morton-Cooper 2000: 14). Waterman et al. (2001) reviewed AR studies in nursing and healthcare and found a 'real-world' focus, which was highly important for researchers, with many projects embedded in practice settings. Waterman et al. (2001) note that such AR studies had a long 'diagnostic' phase, with data collection and reflection on the local situation, and were highly experiential in nature, with practitioners dealing with complex problems and issues. Addressing this complexity was a source of strength in some studies, but it also meant that the projects can be time-consuming and

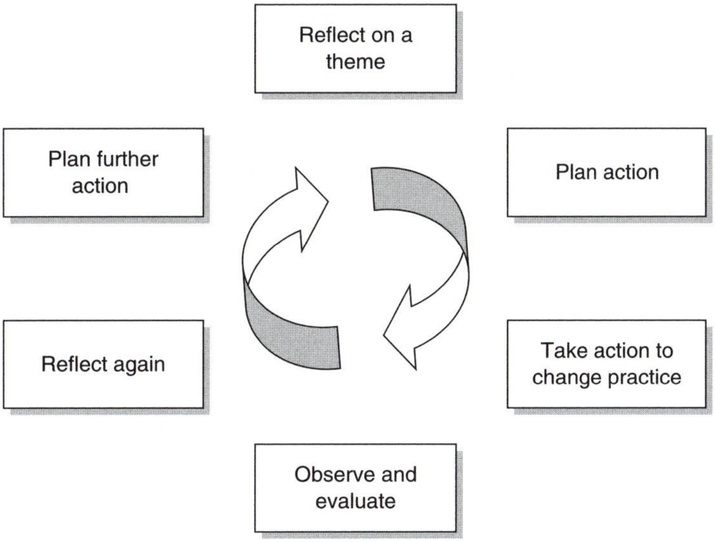

Figure 3.1 Action research spiral with six elements (adapted from Hart and Bond 1995a)

frustrating, highlighting the mismatch between operational policies and the reality of day-to-day life. Success was often difficult to assess due to a lack of precision in defining outcome measures. Greenwood (1994) notes that in healthcare settings, the knock-on effects of changing practice are considerable: when one occupational group jettisons old ways of working, new ways of working may severely challenge other occupational groups. This can alter the status quo and may make effective multidisciplinary working difficult.

Rolfe (1996) discusses how 'traditional' research has largely failed to improve practice because of its embrace of social science research methods, which generate theory without improving conditions for research subjects. Participatory, reflexive and subjective AR methods generate organisational change and close the theory–practice gap (Rolfe 1996). Similarly, Webb (1990) argues that AR has developed in response to the dissatisfaction with traditional research approaches, which change little, and because of their concern to empower people making decisions regarding their own life changes. AR is ideal for healthcare practitioners because it builds on people's motivations, gives them authority and offers support and resources in change processes, and enables them to learn more about research at the same time (Webb 1989).

AR in healthcare settings has four potential benefits (Waterman et al. 2001). These are:

- the development of new services;
- improvements in healthcare, particularly the effectiveness of new policies or untested interventions;

- improvements in the knowledge and understanding of important policy areas among participants; and, increasingly,
- AR projects can be used to secure greater involvement of service users.

Pontin and Lewis (2008) discuss their study, which explored how community children's nurses (CCNs) deliver services to children living with life-limiting, life-threatening and chronic conditions. The researchers were a children's nurse university lecturer, a senior CCN, and 16 CCNs who provide such services. Their aims were to:

- explore ways of managing CCN caseloads to ensure efficiency, effectiveness and equity of service delivery;
- produce an operational caseload management mechanism for CCN teams; and
- produce a mechanism for CCN teams to use in negotiating with agencies/organisations that commission services.

The study generated a number of insights about the sorts of phenomena that contribute to CCNs' perceptions of workload, and in a field where there was little literature they therefore uncovered areas that were hitherto unrecognised in the work of CNNs. Their participants suggested that four themes were important: strategy, being proactive, undertaking purposeful visits, and knowing families. Pontin and Lewis (2008) suggest that CNNs can use their ideas as 'sensitizers' for exploration of their own practice, to work out how they could be proactive in meeting the needs of the families they care for within existing service arrangements, as well as addressing issues of service delivery with commissioners of services.

A further example of how healthcare practice can be changed in real-world healthcare settings is that of Dickinson et al. (2008); two nurses and a research nutritionist. Their action research study was aimed at improving the hospital mealtime experience for older people because poor nutritional care had been a persistent problem. The authors used an action research design, which included role modelling of good practice and critical reflection-in-action on practice. An initial diagnostic phase explored the ward context, using focus groups, interviews, observation and benchmarking. As a result of the study, ward staff felt empowered to make several changes to their nursing practice, including, significantly, that all staff became engaged with, prioritised and were involved in the mealtimes, so that patients were helped effectively with their eating. Dickinson et al. (2008) conclude that their work demonstrates that it is possible to change nursing practice at mealtimes, and that this change can drastically improve patients' in-hospital experience, with all the concomitant benefit accruing from better nutrition, such as improved wound healing and infection recovery rates. In Chapter 4 we discuss further how AR can advance patient care, but also recognise the many challenges that arise when conducting research in the messy real world of practice.

Generating new theory about nursing practice using action research

As well as changing practice, AR has also been used to generate new theory (Holter and Schwartz-Barcott 1993), but this discovery of things or ideas that were previously unknown is not accepted uncritically. Some authors (for example, Titchen and Binnie 1994 and Elliott 2009) argue that the generation of new theory is not a fundamental aim of AR. Rather, it is more about changing practice, and if theory is generated, this is a subordinate aim to improving practice. This makes action research suitable where little is known about a question or problem, provided that researchers adopt an open stance and a long fact-finding diagnostic phase is carried out. AR is thus able to produce tentative explanatory principles to be tested and refined during a project, and about which the researcher must make professional judgements in order to apply them in context. Practice advances by matching appropriate action to accurate diagnosis of the issues at hand.

If change does not occur and practice does not move forward, Titchen and Binnie (1994) argue that the strategy is inappropriate (although this may not be the case with other studies discussed throughout the book); researchers learn from the experience in conjunction with their participants when they reflect together, and another strategy will be tried. For others reading the account, a rich description of the situation is necessary so that the findings can be contextualised and others enabled to decide if the actions are applicable to their own settings. If there are theoretical insights, these are secondary to facilitating change. For practitioners doing AR, there are likely to be difficulties with 'research-thinking' and 'practice-thinking'. These are seen to be incompatible because of the tension between how practitioners respond and react in practice (immediately and fluently), and how they need to respond as researchers (with rigorous analysis of the situation, careful planning and subsequent adherence to the plan).

Titchen and Binnie (1994) argue that in AR, as in nursing practice, it is necessary to be able to 'think on your feet' rather than act as a researcher, and they argue that this demonstrates how theory generation is subordinate to changing practice.

However, theory generation is a crucial aspect of others' AR projects. Walters and East (2001) worked with homeless women in their study, and were drawn into the realities of the women's lives. The researchers' aim was to explore the experiences of the homeless women, and a conceptual model

Table 3.1 A conceptual framework for nurse-led change and development in clinical practice (reproduced with permission from Bellman 2003)

Collaborative Change Agents	Change Process Strategies	Anticipated Outcomes
Insider or Outsider Facilitator *with* Nurses, Managers, Patients/Carers, Health Care Team	Participative Facilitation Personal Enhancement Demonstrable Interpersonal Support Disempowerment Recognition Staff Empowerment	1) Nurse-led, Patient-focused, Creative Change & Development initiatives. 2) Personal, Professional Practice Development.

emerged which improved understanding of the multiple and complex features of women's homelessness. Previous conceptions of homelessness as a critical event are challenged; rather, homelessness is seen as a cyclical process (which the women called 'our cycle') with common and recurring elements. New ideas about services that might make a difference to the women were proposed, with a strong non-professional emphasis, and the women theorised that there should be a new 'Reality Worker' with experience of homelessness who could thus identify and empathise with them. This AR work, then, did not directly change practice but generated theory, and was empowering and supportive to the women participants.

Action research studies have also enabled the development of conceptual models and frameworks. For example, Galvin et al. (1999) note that, while they aimed at collaboration in their AR project developing aspects of primary health nursing practice, this was very difficult to manage and sustain over time. As they were trying to generate theory, gain users' input and develop a new model for teamworking, they found it difficult to set meaningful objectives at the beginning of the project due to these overlapping objectives. However, they were able to generate new ways of working for teamwork in primary health nursing.

A conceptual framework for nurse-led change and development in clinical practice (Bellman 2003) was elicited from two critical action research projects (see Table 3.1). The change process strategies are evident in Chapters 4 and 5.

In summary, action research can enable new knowledge to be uncovered about situations where previously little or nothing had been known. This new knowledge can be theoretical or conceptual, such as in the work of Walters and East (2001), where the need for new services was uncovered, or for Bellman (2003), who developed a conceptual model for changing practice. This conceptual understanding can be used as a driver for change as it informs action researchers' thinking about 'what to do next'.

••• REFLECTIVE ACTIVITY 3.1 REFLECTIVE EXERCISE •••

Think about what Titchen and Binnie (1994) mean by the terms:

- 'research-thinking' and
- 'practice-thinking'.

Write a short paragraph about what each means to you.

- How does each concept differ?
- Can you see areas where they overlap?
- Can you think of ways in which there are conflicts and/or synergies between the two roles (researcher and practitioner)?
- How can you manage these conflicts and synergies in your day-to-day life?

Please do this exercise before reading the forthcoming section entitled 'Methodological implications of research in one's own organisation' (below) as this will inform your subsequent thinking on the issue.

Interpersonal relationships in nursing action research

Several authors discuss the crucial importance of interpersonal relationships in AR where the researcher acts as a change agent. Morton-Cooper (2000) points out that beginning an AR project is similar to taking on new family members. Webb (1989) details her fears and insecurities when trying to initiate change in a clinical setting, and how she worked hard to overcome these with openness and, as an 'outsider', refusal to get involved in the local micro-politics. Hope (1998) discusses the uncertain outcomes of AR projects: researchers simply do not know where they will end up, which may make it a difficult and confusing journey, but one that nurses are well equipped to take because of their well-developed interpersonal skills and openness to others' views. As well as personal relationships, there is a further dimension of complexity.

Methodological implications of research in one's own organisation

Coghlan and Brannick (2010) discuss the methodological implications for researchers working in their own organisations, arguing that one's whole self, rather than a defined part, is caught up in the project. This process will transform the individual, who is required to look at their organisation through fresh eyes and develop new relationships and a new understanding at first hand. Rather than being an outside 'ethnographic' observer, the insider is intimately connected with policies and personalities. This can be useful in the project because the insider does not need to learn new terminologies and ways of working, but it can also be problematic when the researcher encounters the micro-politics of their organisation, particularly if they plan to stay employed there at the end of the project (see also Chapter 4). There is also a dichotomy between the action researcher who adopts the role of project manager for an organisation and the needs of the researcher who may be undertaking research for a higher degree, because the broad criteria for success are different. An organisation is likely to measure success by the extent to which practice is changed or developed, whereas in a higher degree submission, this may be only one of many aspects of the academic quality and rigour of the work. An example of successful project management is discussed in Chapter 5. Yet, the organisational researcher may also work with other participants and develop a range of strategies to effect change but not have authority to implement them, or have more senior colleagues with little detailed understanding of the project work (Coghlan and Brannick 2010).

Coghlan and Brannick (2010) discuss how the knowledge and insights of the insider action researcher relate not only to a theoretical understanding of the organisation, but also to the lived experience of the organisation's dynamics, jargon and taboos (Coghlan 2001). They argue that organisations lead two lives. The formal documentary life of mission statements, policies and procedures may contrast sharply with the informal private life, which individuals and groups experience as cultural norms, traditions and shifting power alliances, love and hate, jealousy and goodwill, infighting, cliques and political factions, and these stand in stark contrast to the rational image which organisations like to exhibit (Coghlan and Brannick 2010). This is an advantage for insider researchers who understand these issues and are able to participate unobtrusively (Coghlan 2001), but is also a disadvantage as they are close to them, and this may hinder the reframing that is necessary for an analysis of events. Thus an insider must work consciously to overcome their pre-understanding and be dispassionate about it when writing an account. This can create tensions between roles which can be difficult to reconcile for action researchers and involves skilled interpersonal communication.

The methodological implications already addressed particularly concern researchers working in their own organisations, and how the day-to-day reality of structures and relationships can influence AR work. Further examples of these kinds of role conflicts and how they were reconciled include Titchen and Binnie's study (1993a). They discuss how they established a 'double-act' relationship in their work developing patient-centred nursing (where Binnie was working in her own organisation) to utilise their complementary interpersonal skills. Despite different professional backgrounds, they shared the same basic values on healthcare and worked collaboratively as 'actor' (facilitator/change agent) and 'researcher'. Titchen and Binnie (1993a, 1993b) note that their model differs from more traditional group models in the AR literature, and rather than trying to work in a 'strictly collaborative manner' (their terminology), they created 'collaborative groups' of ward sisters and staff nurses, then worked with them in their double-act roles to develop nursing practice. The authors reported that this required a great deal of sensitivity in their leadership roles and was demanding and draining, but satisfying overall. However, the 'double-act' role has not always been so successful. In his work as research assistant to an AR project attempting to implement primary nursing, Pontin (Webb et al. 1998) expected to work with an experienced clinical nurse specialist (CNS), who was to be the insider facilitating change. His role was initially about evaluating the initiative, but Pontin experienced considerable ambiguity when appointed as research assistant because the CNS was on long-term sick leave when Pontin arrived, and ward staff looked to him for project management and support. He was keen to become involved with these aspects of the work, but did not have the managerial authority to take them on. When the CNS returned, there was initially a clearer distinction between research and facilitation elements, but with the eventual appointment of a new CNS, Pontin found his roles continually blurred and altered in order to facilitate the project. The fluctuation in the visibility of the CNS meant that he was quickly required to go from being an outsider to an insider. This was confusing for staff as well as stressful for Pontin, who found himself in a different role from that to which he had been appointed. Flexibility and good interpersonal skills are thus essential (see Chapter 4).

Galvin et al.'s (1999) study employed a 'research-practitioner' acting as a change agent to introduce new roles in a district nursing team. They believed that this person could facilitate change by working as part of the nursing team. Continuous negotiation was required between the nurses involved, particularly the research-practitioner's role within the team and her relationships with the clinical nurses, who misinterpreted her function as being primarily part of the nursing workforce. She encountered role confusion and did not meet the expectations of other participants, several of whom found the changes planned for new working practices very challenging. Galvin et al. encountered the resistance to change and abdication of leadership within the clinical team difficult to overcome.

Webb et al. (1998) decided that the action researcher in their study needed to build trust between herself and ward-based staff. The action researcher was an experienced district nurse who had been seconded from her lecturing post by a Health Authority to set up community services for HIV patients. However, at that time, in this particular Health Authority, the majority of AIDS care took place in hospital. Thus the researcher worked as a staff nurse in the unit, but she initially perceived there to be a secretive and protective atmosphere among the nurses. She failed a clinical 'initiation ceremony' involving safety aspects of IV medication administration but, rather than withdrawing from the situation, she persevered and eventually became more accepted by staff, who realised that her goal of establishing community services for this client group was worthwhile. Staff then came to accept her as 'one of the family'. With a grounding in ward-based work, she was able to develop a Community Liaison Team which provided much-needed support for herself, and quickly developed effective community services.

Webb's (1989) strategy in her AR work developing nursing and management skills in a clinical area involved working as a nurse on the chosen ward in order to build rapport with all the ward staff before attempting action or change, and not controlling or dominating clinical situations as a result of her concurrent role as a nurse teacher. Although embarrassing and uncomfortable at first, eventually the strategy enabled her to be accepted as a colleague, established her credibility with the nurses and, as a result, the personal relationships were instrumental in carrying out the project.

Hart and Bond (1995b) outline Bond's involvement in trying to change medication practices in a nursing home. Being the home's manager gave her valuable access to documentation and participants, but she was still severely constrained by lack of time and resources, as she had to continue with the responsibilities of her role. Having responsibility for dispensing medications, she was intimately familiar with the residents' needs, issues of safe dispensing of medication and staff training. However, despite being an insider, she met with considerable resistance to change from senior staff exhibiting poor practice and caring behaviour towards residents, who, she perceived, turned residents' entitlement to medications into a power game, although this resistance was eventually overcome and change in practice occurred.

In summary, the methodological implications of doing AR in one's own organisation centre on three elements: the extent to which the researcher experiences issues of access to personnel and key resources; conflicts in role between that of worker or manager and that of researcher; and the importance of well-developed interpersonal skills and flexibility in overcoming these conflicts.

Participatory action research in healthcare and nursing research: improving 'quality of life' for individuals and communities

Chapter 1 contains material on participatory action research (PAR) , which is identified as a strand of AR with an agenda that seeks to make explicit issues of oppression and to engage in strategies to overcome them. A strand of PAR has emerged in nursing and healthcare research which seeks to 'create knowledge that is necessary for people to take action to improve the quality of their lives' (Koch et al. 2002: 109).

Koch et al. (2002) discuss projects where the PAR approach was used. In their study of workplace violence, critical reflection on nurses' personal experiences was facilitated, and this dialogue was instrumental in the development of a model of best practice and an education package to help nurses deal with violence at work. In a second example, Koch and her participants developed wound management practices, and the collaborative nature of the project not only changed practice, but also benefited group relationships and job satisfaction. A third study empowered women with multiple sclerosis who presented with urinary incontinence to develop self-management techniques. They also petitioned government agencies to improve access to public toilets, and improved the distribution of incontinence supplies by manufacturers.

Koch and Kralik (2006) outline their participatory action research in developing a community health organisational partnership, with the explicit attempt to empower previously disenfranchised people. The written accounts, like all action research, are highly context-specific, where the researcher's task is to facilitate participants' understanding of their situation and how to change it. They give as an example their work with Australian aboriginal elders, in the Eyre Peninsula in South Australia. Their concern was the apparent epidemic of diabetes mellitus among these people, where approximately 200 of the 600-strong community had diabetes and had death rates of over 200% compared to other aboriginal Australians in South Australia. Usual medical management had yielded little success and contemporary reports had called for greater community involvement in their own healthcare. The researchers viewed the issue from a different perspective than that of 'ensuring compliance' to medical treatment, believing instead that skilful facilitation could be used to empower the community to successfully undertake effective diabetes care. As well as working collaboratively to improve diabetes care, the researchers also wanted to leave a legacy of understanding of PAR, which could then be used again as a technique. They met with the community as a whole and then with specific interest groups, such as women, youth clubs, and the elderly. This approach ensured the greatest collaboration from the community. They used a 'Look, Think, Act' methodology (discussed in Chapter 1, and see Figure 1.3), which contained the following elements:

- Look: Participants were encouraged to talk about their experiences of diabetes, focusing on lifestyle issues, life-changing episodes, elements that help successful management, and personal feelings about their illness. Forty contact hours were utilised, and after the initial session the elders set the agenda. This story-telling was immensely powerful as a tool for engagement.

- Think: The group identified four themes that impact on their management of type 2 diabetes. These were nutrition, better understanding of the condition, education for the young, and support for the wider community. These themes were linked with the need to develop a supportive environment. Community members discussed diabetes as something over which they had no control, although as the story-telling progressed participants were able to make the links between alcohol, nutrition, exercise and medication, and lifestyle adjustments were made. The elders were instrumental in this process.
- Act: The elders developed a culture in which the group members felt safe and able to discuss their issues openly. The dominant emotion was fear, which controlled their lives, particularly fear of doctors and of diagnosis. These fears created negative attitudes, depression and a sense of failure. It barred their progress and understanding of the disease, despite the wealth of available resources. Participants believed they would 'just get over it' and did little for themselves to cope with the impact of the illness.

The elders realised that fear was a central issue and as other participants came to realise this too, they moved from fear to courage. This courage was expressed when they became able to accept the diagnosis, and confidence was increased as they realised they were not alone.The group was able to improve its knowledge, which added substantially to the extent of their control and choices about their health. The elders produced a booklet outlining their experiences of diabetes, and discussed their hopes and fears, even taking their knowledge 'on tour' around the community. This health promotion work was liberating, and had a beneficial impact on their community's health development.

PAR methodology has also been used elsewhere to secure community involvement in health promotion projects. Lindsey and McGuinness (1998) discuss work aimed at reducing the risk of falls among older people in Canada, and Lindsey et al. (1999) outline a second project to develop supported living and respite facilities with HIV and AIDS sufferers. In both projects, there is an explicit critical theory perspective, and the researchers argue that PAR enables nurses to create effective partnerships with 'oppressed' groups, with the researcher as a skilled facilitator, as PAR methodology involves community members taking control of change processes and developing leadership roles. Lindsey et al. (1999: 1243) state that 'the knowledge, skills and expertise of nurses engaged in these processes are very different from the more traditional "expert" role of professional practice'. Thus practitioners and researchers must relinquish professional control and trust their participants in the community.

Summary

This chapter has used a number of examples of studies as well as other theoretical material to explore how action research has been applied to nursing and healthcare practice. Examples of how AR can be used for:

- changing practice using action research; and
- generating new theory about practice using action research

have been outlined. In addition, some ideas about the importance of interpersonal relationships in nursing action research have been discussed, as has the importance of an awareness of the action researcher's location within their own organisation (Coghlan and Brannick 2010). PAR has been explored in healthcare and nursing research as one approach for improving 'quality of life' for individuals and communities.

Further reading

Coghlan, D and Brannick, T (2010) *Doing action research in your own organisation* (3rd edition). London: Sage. An excellent text for those within their own organisations.

Glasson, JB, Chang, EML, Bidewell, JW (2008) The value of participatory action research in clinical nursing practice. *International Journal of Nursing Practice* 14: 34–39. Clarifies issues concerning PAR.

Koch, T and Kralik, D (2006) *Participatory action research in healthcare*. Oxford: Blackwell. An excellent text on PAR with lots of experiential material from the authors.

Waterman, HA, Marshall, MN, Noble, J, Davies, H, Walshe, K, Sheaff, R and Elwyn, G (2007) The role of action research in the investigation and diffusion of innovations in health care: The PRIDE project. *Qualitative Health Research* 17(3): 373–381.

Waterman, HA, Tillen, D, Dickson, R and de Koning, K (2001) Action research: A systematic review and assessment for guidance. *Health Technology Assessment* 5(23): 1–166.

Useful websites

Action Research e-reports: www2.fhs.usyd.edu.au/arow/arer/index.html. Lots of resources including methodological hints and tips.

Jean McNiff's website: www.jeanmcniff.com/index.html. Lots of useful resources, mostly from education but with some relevance to healthcare.

Government of Victoria, Australia: www.health.vic.gov.au/healthpromotion. Useful information on health promotion, including some action research studies. Search the site using 'action research'.

Guidelines and Categories for Classifying Participatory Research Projects in Health: www.lgreen.net/guidelines.html. Lots of useful references.

References

Bellman, L (2003) *Nurse-led change and development in clinical practice*. London: Whurr Publishers.

Bridges, J and Meyer, J (2007) Exploring the effectiveness of action research as a tool for organisational change in health care. *Journal of Research in Nursing* 12(4): 389–399.

Coghlan, D (2001) Insider action research projects. *Management Learning* 32(1): 49–60.

Coghlan, D and Brannick, T (2010) *Doing action research in your own organisation* (3rd edition). London: Sage.

Dickinson A, Welch C & Ager L (2008) No longer hungry in hospital: improving the hospital mealtime experience for older people through action research. *Journal of Clinical Nursing* 17, 1492–1502.

Elliott, J (2009) Building educational theory through action research. In Noffke, S E and Somekh, B (eds) (2009), *The Sage handbook of educational action research*. London: Sage, Chapter 1.

Galvin, K, Andrewes, C, Jackson, D, Cheesman, S, Fudge, T, Ferris, R and Graham, I (1999) Investigating change within the primary health care nursing team. *Journal of Advanced Nursing* 30(1): 238–247.

Greenwood, J (1994) Action research: A few details, a caution and something new. *Journal of Advanced Nursing* 20(13): 13–18.

Hart, E (1996) Action research as a professionalising strategy: Issues and dilemmas. *Journal of Advanced Nursing* 23(3): 454–461.

Hart, E and Bond, M (1995a) Developing action research in nursing. *Nurse Researcher* 2(3): 4–14.

Hart, E and Bond, M (1995b) *Action research for health and social care: A guide to practice*. Buckingham: Open University Press.

Holter, I M and Schwartz-Barcott, D (1993) Action research: What is it? How has it been used and how can it be used in nursing? *Journal of Advanced Nursing* 18: 298–304.

Hope, K (1998) Starting out with action research. *Nurse Researcher* 6(2): 16–26.

Koch, T and Kralik, D (2006) *Participatory action research in healthcare*. Oxford. Blackwell.

Koch, T, Selim, P and Kralik, D (2002) Enhancing lives through the development of a community-based participatory action research programme. *Journal of Clinical Nursing* 11(1): 109–117.

Lindsey, E and McGuiness, L (1998) Significant elements of community involvement in participatory action research: Evidence from a community project. *Journal of Advanced Nursing* 28(5): 1106–1114.

Lindsey, E, Shields, L and Stajduhar, K (1999) Creating effective nursing partnerships: Relating community development to participatory action research. *Journal of Advanced Nursing* 29(5): 1238–1245.

Morton-Cooper, A (2000) *Action research in health care*. London: Blackwell Science.

Pontin, D and Lewis, M (2008) Managing the caseload: A qualitative action research study exploring how community children's nurses deliver services to children living with life-limiting, life-threatening and chronic conditions. *Journal for Specialists in Paediatric Nursing* 13(1): 26–35.

Rolfe, G (1996) Going to extremes: Action research, grounded practice and the theory-practice gap in nursing. *Journal of Advanced Nursing* 24(6): 1315–1320.

Titchen, A and Binnie, A (1993a) Research partnerships: Collaborative action research in nursing. *Journal of Advanced Nursing* 18: 858–865.

Titchen, A and Binnie, A (1993b) The 'double act': Co-action researcher roles in an acute hospital setting. In A Titchen and A Binnie, *Changing nursing practice through action research*. Report No.6. Oxford: National Institute for Nursing Centre for Practice Development and Research, Chapter 3.

Titchen, A and Binnie, A (1994) Action research: A strategy for theory generation and testing. *International Journal of Nursing Studies* 31(1): 1–12.

Walters, S and East, L (2001) The cycle of homelessness in the lives of young mothers: The diagnostic phase of an action research project. *Journal of Clinical Nursing* 10(2): 171–179.

Waterman, H, Tillen, D, Dickson, R and de Koning, K (2001) Action research: A systematic review and guidance for assessment. *Health Technology Assessment* 5(23): 1–166. Southampton: The National Coordinating Centre for Health Technology Assessment. Available online at: www.ncchta.org/project/1007.asp (accessed 30/9/2010).

Webb, C (1989) Action research: Philosophy, methods and personal experiences. *Journal of Advanced Nursing* 14: 403–410.

Webb, C (1990) Partners in research. *Nursing Times* 86(32): 40–44.

Webb, C, Turton, P and Pontin, D (1998) Action research: The debate moves on. In B Roe and C Webb (eds), *Research and development in clinical nursing practice*. London: Whurr Publishers, Chapter 14.

4

CLINICAL ACTION RESEARCH TO ADVANCE PATIENT CARE

Loretta Bellman

Healthcare practitioners and academic colleagues have a professional responsibility to contribute to the advancement of patient care. The action research approach is compatible with healthcare professionals' ability to work together, with a common goal of improving patient care. The action research process is akin to the nursing process in that it encompasses identifying and assessing patient-centred problems, action planning, implementing the plan and evaluating the outcomes. It also brings research into the clinical area and enables nurses as a group to actively participate in defining and improving their practice (La Pine 2008).

Chapter objectives

The objectives of this chapter are to:

- provide insight into the role of the clinical action researcher;
- propose practical ways of conducting the action research process with practitioners in clinical settings;
- consider the future for advancing practice-based research and development.

The focus of action research is conducting research *with* rather than *on* people. Achieving meaningful change that benefits patients and enables staff and organisational learning is therefore best managed through the collaboration of frontline staff themselves. It has long been recognised (Toulmin & Gustavsen 1996) that far from the participation of the workers being an obstacle to research – a threat to its objectivity – the most effective way of developing such a project is to enlist into the research procedures the very individuals employed in the institution under investigation. Bate (2000) goes a stage further in believing that it is really about getting people to confront and 'own' their problems, and an invitation for them to become reflective practitioners; and even more than that, to develop a radical critique of their customary ways of working.

A Health Technology Assessment report (Waterman et al. 2001) demonstrated multiple uses of action research to advance patient care:

- for role development;
- contributing to innovation and improvements in healthcare;
- developing knowledge and understanding in practitioners;
- for involvement of patients and NHS staff.

The methodology is also considered appropriate for the implementation of evidence based practice (Munten et al. 2010) and for the integration of patient safety research, healthcare policy and practice (Bellman et al. 2011).

Collaborative engagement in a practice-based research project, from project identification to outcome evaluation, is both exciting and challenging. It is evident that engaging with colleagues to undertake an action research project in the messy real world of practice is both a demanding journey and a grand adventure (La Pine 2008). There is fundamental recognition that the ability of the action researcher, an organisation's culture, support at a senior level, and the clinical setting or context, will affect the chances of completing the study. Whilst this may appear obvious to some, this chapter provides practical advice from the literature in a range of care settings, and from personal experience, for increasing the likelihood of success of a clinical action research project. Academic support can also enhance the likelihood of achieving innovative patient-centred outcomes. The practitioner and academic may adopt either the role of action research facilitator or that of co-researcher. Basically if you get your head around action research and how to go about it, get appropriate support and take it carefully, it is achievable and a great way to look at and improve practice.

Self preparation

Adopting the role of clinical action researcher is comparable to being a clinical change agent and a contemporary leader, the focus of which is collaboration (Archer & Cameron 2009). A key factor is the ability to collaborate across boundaries to facilitate colleagues in researching practice (see Chapter 6). Wherever you choose to place yourself on a novice-expert research continuum, identifying your personal and professional transferable skills can be very useful prior to leading and facilitating a clinical action research project. Good preparation also includes critical analysis of past action research studies to provide insight and understanding.

••• REFLECTIVE ACTIVITY 4.1 •••

Reflect on action research literature that you have read and identify your transferable skills for leading and facilitating a clinical action research project.

Transferable skills for clinical action research include: personal insight and self-awareness; confidence in communicating at different levels within the organisation; a flexible approach; realistic time-keeping; effective collaborator; understanding colleagues' clinical pressures and workload; demonstrating sensitivity to the emotional needs, work and social demands of colleagues. A fundamental knowledge of action research is required (see Chapters 1–3). Although the literature clearly demonstrates that every action research project is unique, transferable knowledge from one action research project can inform the next. Gaining understanding of the following is also recommended:

- organisational culture;
- strategic *and* operational change management approaches;
- political acumen and leadership;
- transformational leadership;
- theories of reflection;
- project management;
- practice development;
- process consultancy;
- espoused theory & theory-in-action (Argyris & Schön 1974);
- the concepts of collaboration, facilitation, negotiation, power, empowerment, influence, resilience and conflict resolution.

Insider or outsider?

The literature implies that there is more likelihood of a successful outcome if the action researcher is an insider (Coghlan & Brannick 2010; Williams et al 2008). An insider action researcher may believe that they know many of the strengths, weaknesses, opportunities and threats that currently exist in their practice setting and organisation. This perspective is challenged by a number of authors. For example, a change in a familiar context can be challenging as Meyer (1995) found with the arrival of a new manager in a ward where her patient involvement study was being undertaken, which made her feel like an 'outsider'. For La Pine (2008), her experience and knowledge in intensive care nursing made her ideally positioned to undertake action research in practice. Yet, on moving from a staff nurse post in the unit to that of Research Coordinator (a positive move), she saw herself as neither insider nor outsider but as being able to walk in both worlds (Bonner & Tolhurst 2002).

For action researchers who are external to an organisation, different approaches to how best to engage with potential research participants have to be considered. For example, access for Hockley (2006) involved an exploratory phase in which she worked early shifts, late shifts and night shifts in order to get to know staff and for them to get to know her. I was granted access to implement the findings from a phenomenological study which recommended a follow-up action research project for change and development in a day surgery unit (Bellman 2003). Part of the critical reflexive account is to be found in Box 4.1.

Box 4.1

Part of a critical reflexive account of an outsider clinical action researcher (Bellman 2003: 235)

Facilitating the first meeting with the co-researchers resulted in a positive outcome. Whilst I felt disadvantaged as an outsider I also recognised that this was advantageous in establishing a rapport with the co-researchers. By requesting knowledge of the organisation and of the clinical context, the co-researchers were able to share factual information as well as their personal insights. This strategy began the process of collaborative practice, particularly as two of the co-researchers had not previously met.

However, the open dialogue that I tried to promote no doubt disturbed a carefully controlled social environment. It also appeared to have disturbed micro political alignments and challenge individual positions of power and influence. As an outsider my initial entry into the organisation reflected Stringer's (1996) advice, to be 'as "soft" as possible'. The approach to managers, the ethics committee, and my engagement with the staff was candid and non-confrontational.

Consideration of the needs of the outsider action researcher is necessary due to the increase in cross boundary working, the growth of partnership organisations, and organisational recognition of the advantages of collaboration. Whether you perceive yourself to be an insider or outsider action researcher (or indeed both), undertaking a clinical action research project requires you to adopt a pragmatic and flexible way of working, particularly when seeking managerial support.

Engaging managerial support

Justifying to managers the need for an action research project with staff engagement in working hours can be challenging. Whilst it can be argued that developing practice through clinical action research is an essential element of improving care for patients, some may perceive it as a 'luxury' and not a necessity. Sources of funding for action research, for example to backfill an action researcher or co-researchers' time, are very much in the minority. Strategies for overcoming managerial resistance and eliciting political support are proposed (Roth et al 2007):

- Anchor the project in the organisation and find the right stakeholders and sponsors at all levels of the organisation, including whenever possible patients/carers;
- Be 'street smart' and know how to get things done;
- Work in collaboration with influential others to move the project forward;
- Try to ensure that the first interventions and change in the project have a wide impact on a wide range of organisational members.

It is also recommended that you:

- identify an influential champion at a senior level in the organisation;
- disseminate the project proposal and developments in a user-friendly format via electronic, written and oral accounts to all levels of the organisation (see Chapter 8);
- try to position the project so that it has widespread buy-in and ownership and a formal line of reporting instead of sitting in isolation;
- be alert to and confront saboteurs who try to subvert, obstruct, disrupt the project. They may try to conceal their identities because of the consequences of their actions.

••• REFLECTIVE ACTIVITY 4.2 •••

Consider ways in which you can try to overcome managerial resistance and achieve support within the organisation.

Energy, commitment, passion and political skill are all required. Political skills include the lobbying process (Box 4.2) which can prove most useful in both gaining and then sustaining support for a study. All skills take time to learn and require practice.

Box 4.2

Lobbying skills (adapted from Wingfield 2008)

- Understand who the key stakeholders are and know what is on their agenda;
- Understand the local politics of your area and the national health care political agenda;
- Preparation – do your homework, have evidence, use facts, figures and patient stories to support your argument;
- Communicate in a succinct, calm, confident, positive manner;
- Be passionate about the focus of the project;
- Be respected in your specialist field.

• • • REFLECTIVE ACTIVITY 4.3 • • •

To what extent do you meet the criteria identified in Box 4.2? How will you address your skills gap? What else could you do to enlist political support?

Identifying the project

How do you identify the research objective(s) or research question(s)? You may have an idea of the issue or innovation you wish to study. As the focus of clinical action research is collaborative change and development you will need to explore what you *and* front-line colleagues wish to change in a clinical setting. The focus for change may be recognised at the start of a project. However, it may not be until the project is underway that you as action researcher with colleagues, often called co-researchers, focus on specific objectives or identify specific research questions. As Streubert Speziale & Carpenter (2007: 335) highlight, the nurse researcher who chooses action research has to be comfortable with 'others' making the decision about what is best for them. Equally, a clinical manager can have difficulty acknowledging their staff's ownership of a project:

> 'I know that initially it was quite difficult for me. I wanted to come up with some of my ideas, but then I took a step back and thought you know what it is about, it has got to be from them and whatever will come will be of benefit. I can remember feeling a little bit aggrieved, I wish I could do what I want to.' (Nurse Unit Manager, in Bellman 2003:137)

Ways to gain management support in the clinical setting include:

- demonstrating how the project has direct links to national and local healthcare policy;

- describing an 'action research' project as a clinical change programme, as the term is controversial (see Chapter 3) and not always clearly understood in healthcare organisations;
- openly acknowledging that patients' needs remain the priority rather than the project. Anticipate that at times co-researcher clinical workload may delay project development with them;
- link the project to delivering key organisational imperatives.

Patient involvement

Patient and carer involvement is gaining impetus in healthcare research although, according to a systematic review of published nursing action research studies (Munn-Giddings et al. 2008), only a small number of patients or carers have been research participants. Engaging with patients and carers as co-participants at different stages of a project, or as co-researchers throughout a project, has significant benefits. For Elsey & Lathlean (2006) involving service users/patients as co-researchers was beneficial in challenging professional viewpoints and offering alternative perspectives. Parents of people with intellectual disabilities were co-researchers in the study by Walmsley & Mannan (2009). Schipper et al. (2010) describe a patient researcher's reflections on how the project contributed to her empowerment, engendered feelings of pride and self-confidence regarding her experiential knowledge, and how it changed her relationship with her disease. Also, committees were willing to support and sustain the project because of the clear involvement of patients as research partners.

Project overview

Ensuring a clear audit trail is the responsibility of the action researcher. An audit trail is a transparent description of the research steps taken from the start of a research project to the development and reporting of findings (Cohen & Crabtree 2006). The audit trail includes: how the project was initiated; engagement of co-researchers; collaborative reflection on practice and reaching consensus on the identification of the patient-centred issue, action planning, implementation, reflection and evaluation of the change process. The seven criteria, as delineated by Hart & Bond (1995; 37–38) guide the action research process:

Action Research

1 is educative;
2 deals with individuals as members of social groups;
3 is problem-focused, context-specific and future-oriented;
4 involves a change intervention;
5 aims at improvement and involvement;
6 involves a cyclic process in which research, action and evaluation are interlinked;
7 is founded on a research relationship in which those involved are participants in the change process.

An additional criterion is recommended for clinical action research – project preparation and assessment:

8 exposes dimensions of organisational culture, power and control.

Project preparation and assessment

There is much to consider in the preparatory and assessment stage of a clinical action research project. Preparation includes assessing: key stakeholders' views of, and commitment to, an action research project; managers' support for the project and timeline; the motivation of the co-researchers, their understanding of the action research process and their participation in developing the project timeline; accessing a quiet room for co-researcher meetings, and identifying colleagues to provide support. The following prerequisites to project implementation are considered essential:

- Discuss the project and nature of action research with key stakeholders and, at the same time, establish your credibility to undertake the study;
- Stress the preference for voluntary participation of staff co-researchers rather than manager selection, and agree dates with the manager for regular feedback of project progress;
- Negotiate protected time for ongoing co-researcher review meetings;
- Ensure a physically comfortable environment for the co-researchers' meetings to enable them to have a 'safe communicative space';
- Explain to the co-researchers the ongoing consent process during project development and obtain their written consent to participate (see chapter 7);
- Establish a realistic project timeline with all the co-researchers;
- Establish a steering/advisory Group to include a funder representative, especially if receiving external funding, to share actions and concerns;

- Devise a communication strategy to ensure all co-researchers are kept up to date with the project in spite of ill health, annual leave, and unavoidable non-attendance at planned co-researcher meetings;
- Identify appropriate colleagues to provide clinical, academic, and emotional support.

Ensuring a communicative space

It is highly unlikely that a project will succeed without both the manager's commitment to protected time for the co-researchers and the commitment of the co-researchers to attend their regular meetings and engage in a 'communicative space'. The success or failure of an action research venture may depend on what happens at the beginning of the enquiry process: in the way access is established, and on how participants and co-researchers are engaged early on (Wicks & Reason 2009). The first step in action research turns out to be central: the formation of a 'communicative space' in a way that articulates an issue of concern, allows participants to voice divergent views in a democratic context, permits the mutual understanding and the evolution of new practices which arise and are tested through authentic engagement (Carr & Kemmis 1986).

The safe communication space enables the action researcher and co-researchers to share their knowledge and experience in a mutually supportive environment and also to expose their lack of knowledge and expertise, without embarrassment or fear of intimidation. Anticipating and addressing the emotional, task and organisational issues of the co-researchers is a key strategy for the action researcher – initially for establishing a communicative space, and latterly for ongoing review during the change process. Addressing the questions in Box 4.3 are useful first steps.

Box 4.3

Co-researchers' emotional, task & organisational issues (Wicks & Reason 2009)

Emotional issues

Who will I be in this group?
Will I belong?

Task issues

Will this group meet my needs?
Will I be able to contribute?
Will we be free to follow our own purposes?

Organisational issues

How much time will I have to spend on the project?
Can I fit it into my busy schedule?
How does it 'fit' within my everyday work activities?

Both drivers and barriers to change are reflected upon and the action researcher needs to anticipate, manage and contain both group and individual anxiety, particularly around unwelcome truths (Spalding 2009). For example, within the development of a new nursing role (Bellman & Corrigan 2010) co-researchers identified a 'rollercoaster of emotions' reflecting role ambiguity and role conflict. An ongoing system of support that they valued within the communicative space was group reflection on their experiences. They also shared aspects of their individual clinical supervision, negotiated and undertaken with a chosen senior clinical colleague who worked in the hospital but was external to the project. As the project progressed, the findings from focus groups with ward staff included support for the new role, and colleagues' recognition of the co-researchers' commitment to improving patient care, their new knowledge and improved changes in patient care.

The timeline

The clinical context requires the action researcher to work within the limitations of colleagues by co-ordinating the research project and by being efficient with their time (Spalding 2009). Even with these considerations, slippage of the project timeline can and does occur. Anticipate that there may be a delay in receiving ethical clearance (see Chapter 7). Co-researcher meetings may have to be rescheduled due to heavy workload, staff shortages, co-researcher annual leave, and ill health.

Fundamental to project development is the ability of the action researcher to negotiate with managers and co-researchers a realistic timeline, to develop it together and to have it on display. Regular co-researcher meetings, every 2–4 weeks, are the prime consideration. Always overestimate the time required for each stage of the project, even when the focus of the project has been agreed. Working backwards from the anticipated completion date can be useful.

If planning to conduct face-to-face interviews, telephone interviews or focus groups always err on the side of caution. Be as accommodating as possible regarding date and time to meet, length of meeting, and venue. Even with these preparations the demands on participants, particularly practitioners, are such that they may not be able to attend. Be as flexible as possible and plan to have back-up dates included in the timeline whenever possible.

The direction of travel of the project may not always be clear and learning to live with ambiguity (for longer periods of time than anticipated) is a common occurrence for the action researcher. Reflecting on the positive outcomes of their Dignity and Respect project, Crow et al. (2009) assert that inevitably action research takes on a life of its own, and it can be difficult to pre-empt the development of the project.

Support

Meyer (1993) refers to the action researcher's extreme isolation and self-doubt which is aggravated by having to learn to develop methods and strategies in the field (unlike most research which can be planned in advance). Not all action researchers will have identified the need for support but it is strongly recommended. A trusted colleague or formal clinical supervisor will listen, offer encouragement and explore challenges and options throughout the research journey. Even those with a research supervisor embedded in action research may also choose to have colleague support. Maintaining a confidential reflective journal is an essential research method in action research but also a source of support. Writing down project achievements, however small, on a regular basis, and the challenges of change, can be experienced as a therapeutic process.

• • • REFLECTIVE ACTIVITY 4.4 • • •

Consider your need for support. Identify the most appropriate colleagues to offer you academic, clinical and emotional support.

Project planning and development

The project planning and development stage encompasses the participative facilitation process (see Chapter 6). The action researcher facilitator and co-researchers together: identify/seek evidence for the focus of the project by reflecting on their shared caring values and beliefs, patient care issues, and healthcare literature which can include relevant policy documents. Together they can also identify the research participants; familiarise themselves with the ethical review process; develop research information and consent forms for participants; design and test research tools as appropriate; explore the need for an individual journal to record personal project involvement, and review the project timeline. Consequently the following actions are recommended:

- facilitate the co-researchers' reflection on patient care issues, ensuring sufficient time to identify congruent shared values and beliefs including your own, regarding patient care (see Chapter 6);
- together explore local policy issues and evidence-*informed* practice which encompasses research findings, practice wisdom and service user views (Eccles 2009), to inform decision-making and consensual agreement of the proposed change (see Chapter 6). Being involved in the decision-making process provides an incentive to actively implement change (Glasson et al. 2006);
- appreciate that although exploring one issue at any one time has been recommended (Elliott 1991; Webb 1989), this may in fact delay multiple improvements (Spalding 2009; Bellman 2003);
- encourage co-researcher contribution in: developing the ethics proposal; identifying participants; developing both participant project information and participant consent forms; undertaking literature searches; identifying research methods; developing data collection tools;
- explore with co-researchers their views of recording their participation in a personal reflective journal;
- ensure ongoing review of the timeline.

The exploratory nature of action research is considered creative, innovative and empowering for both action researcher and co-researchers. The approach is underpinned by the values and beliefs of the participants, identification of patient care issues, and support for change and development within the organisation. La Pine (2008), in what she terms the 'reconnaissance phase' or 'engagement phase', of her critical action research study, explored with nurse participants their core values and ideals regarding, in this context, intensive care nursing. The questions that she posed were: What are your own values and beliefs in caring for patients in the Intensive Care Unit? What is your philosophy of nursing? How would you care for your patient if there was no-one to tell you what to do and you did not have to consider anyone else but your patient? The responses enabled La Pine to facilitate a consensus regarding the focus of the action study about which it appeared was somewhat different from her own original idea. Chapter 6 provides further information in reaching a consensus.

Once the focus of the project has been identified, learning how to research together is an ongoing process. Co-researcher participation is to be encouraged at all stages of the research process whilst recognising workload demands.

The eight co-researchers who participated with me in the development of a new nursing role (Bellman & Corrigan 2010) were the Consultant Nurse (cardiac care); the Clinical Nurse Specialist (thoracic care); the Ward Sister (cardiothoracic ward); two Clinical Practice Facilitators and three Staff Nurses who were adopting the new role in turn. Examples of co-researcher project development included:

- Consultant Nurse with one of the Clinical Practice Facilitators helped to develop the ethics proposal;
- all co-researchers identified project participants and participated in developing both project information and consent forms for staff and patients;
- the Clinical Nurse Specialist with one of the Clinical Practice Facilitators undertook a literature search of new nursing role implementation, and action research in nursing;
- all co-researchers participated in identifying the research methods;
- both Clinical Practice Facilitators led on the development of the electronic staff survey tool (Box 4.4); all co-researchers helped to develop the focus group proforma (Box 4.5); the Clinical Nurse Specialist led the development of the patient survey (Box 4.6);
- the ward sister reviewed the original timeline and produced an updated version for each of us.

It was the first time that these clinical staff had been involved in a practice-based research project. They mostly viewed research as distant and elitist bearing little relationship to clinical practice. Research became meaningful with ownership of, and participation in, the project.

Box 4.4

Electronic staff survey tool developed by the Clinical Practice Facilitator co-researchers

Staff 'Perceptions & Expectations' questionnaire

(Electronic version 2)

An increasing number of thoracic patients requiring surgery are being cared for at X Hospital. Thoracic patients have complex needs and it is anticipated that the development of a Thoracic Support Nurse (TSN) role will lead to an improvement in patient care and a potential reduction in in-patient length of stay.

This survey has been developed as part of an Action Research study to inform Thoracic Support Nurse role development. Your contribution to the development and advancement of the role would be much appreciated. The following survey contains six questions and should take approximately 10–15 minutes to complete. All contributions will be anonymous.

1 What are the key issues for you regarding the nursing care of thoracic patients?
2 What do you see as the advantages of the Thoracic Support Nurse role:

- for patients?
- for you?
- for the inter-professional team?
- for the organisation?

3 What do you see as the disadvantages of the Thoracic Support Nurse role:

- for patients?
- for you?
- for the inter-professional team?
- for the organisation?

4 How would you like to see the role develop in the future?
5 Could you see yourself in a Thoracic Support Nurse role? (nurses only)

Yes/No
Why/why not?

6 Anything else you would like to say?

Box 4.5

Focus group proforma

Focus group themes

Preliminary preparation

Ensure:

- a quiet, private environment for up to 10 participants
- all participation is voluntary
- all participants have signed an informed consent form and understand the purpose of the focus group and the focus group process and outcome
- all participants are comfortable with being recorded; if not notes will be taken
- all participants have an equal opportunity to contribute to the focus group.

Themes

The four themes to be addressed are:

- Perceptions of the role – personal, patients, colleagues
- Uniqueness of the role – differences, advantages, disadvantages
- The change process – the barriers and drivers regarding role development
- Future development – issues to be addressed; raising the profile of the role for patients, nursing and multiprofessional colleagues; prioritising future action.

Questions that will be asked:

- Which aspects of the Thoracic Support Nurse role do you value?
- How do patients view the role?

(Continued)

(Continued)

- How do colleagues view the role?
- What is unique/different about the role?
- What are the advantages/disadvantages of the role?
- What is helping to develop the role?
- What is hindering development of the role?
- How would you like to see the role develop in the future?

Prompts that may be used include:

- That's an interesting point, please tell us more.
- Can you say why?
- Is that a shared view?
- What evidence do you have for saying that?
- Is everyone in agreement?
- Can you please clarify?
- Is that an issue for everyone?

Box 4.6

Patient survey tool developed by the Clinical Nurse Specialist co-researcher

Thoracic Support Nurse patient survey

When you were a patient at this hospital you may have received care from the Thoracic Support Nurse. If you did receive care from her your views on this new nurse role will be very welcome. The nurse giving you this form in the outpatients department will firstly ensure that you previously signed a consent form to participate in this research project when you were in hospital. Your views will contribute to developing the role and further improvement of care for patients with chest disorders.

Instructions

Please answer each of these questions by putting a circle around either the **Yes** or the **No** box.

1 When you were admitted to the hospital, were you told that there was a Thoracic Support Nurse?

Yes
No

2 Did you meet the Thoracic Support Nurse during your stay in hospital?

Yes
No

If **No**, thank you for your time. There is no need to complete the form.

3 If **Yes**, you may remember the name of the Thoracic Support Nurse:

The name of the Thoracic Support Nurse is..

4 Did the Thoracic Support Nurse tell you about her role?

Yes
No

5 Did the Thoracic Support Nurse spend enough time with you to meet your needs?

Yes
No

If **NO**, please say which needs were unmet.

6 Did the Thoracic Support Nurse provide enough verbal information about your surgery?

Yes
No

7 Did the Thoracic Support Nurse provide enough written information about your surgery?

Yes
No

8 Did the Thoracic Support Nurse provide you with sufficient information and advice to improve your health in a way you could understand?

Yes
No

9 Did the Thoracic Support Nurse tell you the name of your key worker?

Yes
No

10 Did the Thoracic Support Nurse discuss the follow-up care that you would need when you left hospital?

Yes
No

11 Did you have any contact with the Thoracic Support Nurse after your were discharged from hospital?

Yes
No

Thank you for completing the survey.

••• REFLECTIVE ACTIVITY 4.5 •••

In what ways can you engage your co-researchers in the development phase of your action research project?

Project implementation

Implementing collaborative change in a dynamic clinical context can be seen as a complex intervention process. In this stage of the project it is essential to build confidence in the co-researchers' ability to undertake data collection. The initial phase of data collection is often to gauge colleagues' and patients' perceptions of the proposed change. Prior to implementing the data collection process, discussing and practising interview technique or running a focus group for example, and use of an audio-tape, can all be undertaken within the co-researcher meetings. When and how to implement the change must also be carefully planned. Demonstrable interpersonal support (Bellman 2003) is fundamental during this time, through:

- facilitating co-researcher ongoing reflection on the implementation of the data collection process;
- encouraging feelings of empowerment to be aired and exploring issues of disempowerment, including your own;
- engaging co-researchers in the data analysis process as they wish;
- discussing and using findings from the data to move the project forward;
- agreeing how to address concerns as they occur to enable the co-researchers to be proactive, influence decision-making and feel empowered to challenge and change practice;
- encouraging the co-researchers to identify positive strategies to overcome perceived conflict and reticence to change;
- sustaining own and co-researcher motivation especially when there is slippage of timelines, as is often the case with action research projects conducted in dynamic clinical settings;
- celebrating project milestones.

The importance of facilitating dialogue and shared understanding throughout the project is fundamental to both the change process and sustaining the project (Hockley 2006; Bellman 2003). However, sometimes discussion in clinical settings may have to be brought to a premature close due to the co-researchers' work demands as well as the pressure to act or move the project forward. These practical constraints could impact on understanding one another's point of view, but the thing that holds a group together is tacit or explicit agreement to continue despite the limits and interruptions (Kemmis 2006).

This phase can often be exhilarating and challenging as staff start to experience the potential for, and effects of, clinical change. Time spent preparing clinical staff for the change, preferably in the co-researchers' practice setting, is essential. It is hoped that colleagues will welcome change and be supportive. In an evaluation of a model of nursing care for older patients (Glasson et al. 2006), time constraints and fluctuating nursing staff levels had a contextual impact on project completion. However, Spalding (2009) found, in her study to improve a preoperative education programme for patients awaiting a total hip replacement, that despite being busy participants attended every meeting, demonstrating their commitment to the research. However, the challenges which can arise often reflect the contextual barriers to using and doing research in clinical practice identified by Carlson & Plonczynski (2008), Box 4.7.

Box 4.7

Contextual barriers to using and doing research in clinical practice (adapted from Carlson & Plonczynski 2008)

Contextual barriers

- Insufficient time to implement new ideas
- Lack of staff support
- No time to read research
- Inadequate facilities for implementation
- Physician non-co-operation
- Lack of authority to change
- Withdrawal of support by senior management

According to Coghlan & Casey (2001), probably the most important issue for nurse action researchers, particularly when they want to remain and progress in the hospital, is managing organisational politics. An action research project may be threatening to existing organisational norms, particularly in those organisations that lean towards hierarchal control (Coghlan & Brannick 2010) and a closed communication culture (Hockley 2006). For example: in a study of a new role – the Inter-Professional Care Co-ordinator (Bridges & Meyer 2007), local service managers were both involved in, and supported, the action research project. However, a hierarchal mode of governance was exhibited by the Hospital Trust Board, with 'top down' decision making and where service manager contributions were not valued.

Disempowering issues for the action researcher and co-researchers have to be recorded and ways to resolve them agreed within the regular review meetings. Some of my experiences have included:

- a senior nurse manager's indifference to her staff's creative ideas for patient-centred change and development;
- overt devaluing of an experienced senior nurse's advice by a junior doctor;
- withdrawal of a clinical manager co-researcher from the project;
- no participant attendance at planned focus group meetings;
- refusal by corporate management to continue with a project (Box 4.8).

Box 4.8

Co-facilitators' reaction to senior management's decision to withdraw support for their action research project (Bellman et al. 2003: 192–193)

'But you don't empower people and then disempower them ... in some ways it's very disconcerting and quite ruthless to do that and it isn't how you go about raising morale, standards and enhancing the quality of care. All these things are the aims of the hospital now and certainly come from Government policy in relation to clinical governance and evidence based practice, so it's really mixed messages.' Co-facilitator 1

'What really concerns me about the whole thing is whether they [corporate management] have any moral obligation ... if you actually give someone the chance for self-development, to start a project, and then pull the rug [sic] ... what is the thinking behind that? They can't ignore the fact that what you're doing is changing yourself, changing your practice, changing the organisational culture.' Co-facilitator 2

Hockley (2006: 177) was told by one of the nursing home owners in her study that she might pose a threat to the nurse manager. She reflected on the fact that as a first time action researcher:

> 'I never saw myself as a powerful person – many times, going to the nursing homes, I would feel extremely nervous. I had seen the owners and nurse manager as all-powerful and very much 'in charge'. I now realised that the nurse manager might be more threatened by new things than I had first realised.'

La Pine (2008) recognised that conducting a critical action research project in the area in which she worked proved to be the beginning of a process of self and collective understanding of Intensive Care Unit nursing practice and its relationship with social, economic, legal and political aspects of healthcare. Her project highlighted concerns about conducting action research in her own area of work and what could be construed as political, subversive action (Kemmis, 1993; Williamson & Prosser, 2002). However, the research process enabled the nurses to participate in defining and examining these issues and work together to find solutions.

On many occasions in clinical practice settings, different people, with different goals and needs, may come into conflict. Negative outcomes including personal animosity and strained work relationships can result. Yet, conflict is not necessarily a bad thing. It can lead to personal and professional growth as long as it is resolved effectively. Ways in which this may be achieved include the following.

- Make sure that good relations are the first priority. Remain calm and courteous to one another and remain constructive under pressure.
- Keep people and problems separate. Recognise that in many cases the other person is not just 'being difficult' – real and valid differences can lie behind conflictive positions.
- Pay attention by active listening to the interests that are being presented. Listen first, talk second.
- Set out the 'facts'. Agree and establish the objective, observable elements that will have an impact on the decision.
- Explore options together. Be open to the idea that a third position may exist, and that you can get to your idea jointly. (MindTools.com 2010).

• • • REFLECTIVE ACTIVITY 4.6 • • •

Consider how you would address the barriers to project implementation identified in Box 4.7.

Project process and outcome evaluation

Both process and outcome evaluation are fundamental to an action research project. Quality indicators (see Chapter 10) can inform the evaluation process.

Four key objectives of ongoing process evaluation are to:

- determine how the project is being developed;
- identify drivers and barriers to change and development;
- determine the impact of, and any changes to, the focus of the project;
- review the implementation of proposed solutions to identified problems.

Process evaluation is generally undertaken at the start of each co-researcher meeting. Evidence for the direction of travel of the project will be recorded, in writing and/or audio-taped, from co-researcher feedback and, at certain stages of the project, from data analysis. Process evaluation is guided by the research questions/objectives of the project and questions such as: How is change happening in this clinical setting? Who and what is driving the change forward? Who and what are the barriers to change? To what extent is service user and carer participation evident? Have problems been resolved? How is the action researcher enabling: staff empowerment; disempowerment recognition; facilitative participation; demonstrable interpersonal support, and self-enhancement through learning and increased self-confidence?

Data analysis of, for example, interviews, focus groups, surveys, co-researcher meetings, reflective journals, and emails, all contribute to process evaluation. Depending on the choice of research tools the data analysis process will be either qualitative or quantitative, or both. The key findings or themes that emerge from process evaluation may also reflect outcome evaluation. Outcome evaluation is undertaken at the completion of a project and/or as the action researcher withdraws from the project. Evaluation of patient-centred change includes the unique meaning of the experience for each person. Box 4.9 is one example of an outcome evaluation tool for co-researchers, used for either individual or group interview. Depending on the project, the outcomes of an action research study can be identified and explored with patients, co-researchers, practitioners and the multidisciplinary team of the clinical area, strategic and operational managers and other key stakeholders. Recommended actions include:

- evaluate the extent to which the project's objectives or research questions have been achieved from the perspectives of the co-researchers', participant stakeholders, and action researcher;
- identify with the co-researchers their personal growth and new practice knowledge from participating in the action research process;
- celebrate success;
- ensure action researcher critical reflexivity – the process of considering how your own actions, assumptions, beliefs and values have affected the situation and its interpretation (Porter 1996);
- establish with managers how to sustain and continuously review the change in practice;
- engage co-researchers, if they wish, in co-writing the research report, publication in a peer-reviewed journal, internal and conference presentations.

Many action research projects demonstrate positive outcomes for patients, participants, and the organisation, but not all projects achieve these outcomes or even reach completion. Some projects struggle to reach fruition or achieve what may be perceived as a successful outcome. When a project is incomplete a sense of disappointment, feelings of disempowerment and regret at having let down ones' colleagues is understandable. Yet, much learning results, including greater understanding of the change process. To increase the knowledge base for professional change and development it is equally important to analyse and publish the reasons for non-completion of action research projects as it is to publish results of successful ones.

Box 4.9

Example of an outcome evaluation tool

Outcome evaluation

1 What have you learnt personally and professionally from being a co-researcher in this project?
2 What do you believe overall helped to drive the project forward?
3 What do you consider overall were the barriers to change regarding this project?
4 How were problems resolved?
5 What changes have occurred as a direct result (impact) of the project – for patients/colleagues/multidisciplinary team/the ward/yourself?
6 What could be shared with other colleagues thinking of making a similar change in practice?
7 What could be shared with other colleagues thinking of doing an action research project?
8 How would you like this initiative to continue in the future?
9 Anything else you would like to say?

Evaluation based on:

A The aim of the project is the development of a Thoracic Support Nurse (TSN) role. The objectives are to systematically:

1 explore the process of change with the TSN and colleagues
2 highlight the drivers and barriers to developing the TSN role
3 explore problems within TSN role development
4 evaluate the impact of the TSN role.

B The criteria which distinguish action research from other methodologies include:

- a problem-focused, context-specific and future-oriented approach;
- a change intervention aimed at improvement and involvement;
- those involved are participants/co-researchers in the change process;
- a cyclic process in which research, action and evaluation are interlinked;
- educative for all (Hart & Bond 1995);
- exposes dimensions of organisational culture, power and control (Bellman 2003).

C Herr and Anderson (2005) suggest five quality indicators for action research:

- outcome validity: the extent to which actions address the aims/objectives of the project;
- process validity: the extent to which problems are framed and solved in a way that enables ongoing learning;
- democratic validity: the extent to which research is done in collaboration with all stakeholders;
- catalytic validity: the extent to which the research process reorients, focuses and energises participants towards knowing reality in order to transform it ;
- dialogic validity: peer review.

••• REFLECTIVE ACTIVITY 4.7 •••

Once completed, in what ways can the outcomes of the clinical action research project be sustained?

Published action research projects rarely refer to sustainability or development. Depending on the change in practice, an audit tool or clinical guidelines can be produced to sustain the outcome of the project. Funding for printing patient information leaflets and supporting patient-centred education programmes may be required. For Hockley (2006), an Integrated Care Pathway, for the last days of life, was developed. For a new clinical role that has been successfully implemented and evaluated, a funding commitment for the post plus a job specification are fundamental requirements.

Advancing practice-based research

Both national and local strong leadership is now required to create a clinical academic culture in which to advance practice-based research for patient benefit in diverse clinical settings. The issues regarding the need for a research culture, demonstrating management and medical support, is well rehearsed in the literature (for example Woodward et al. 2007). There is a need for both recognition of applied research projects for patient benefit in local clinical settings and growing support for the concept of evidence-*informed* practice which encompasses research findings, practice wisdom and service user views (Eccles 2009).

Box 4.7 was a useful starting point for the assessment phase of a critical action research project conducted in a UK Hospital Foundation Trust, which provided evidence for a change in regard to nursing and midwifery research and development (Bellman and Wiseman 2010). The co-researchers were Consultant Nurses and the Consultant Midwife, clinical leaders in their field of practice. All are Masters-level prepared, one has a doctorate. Nurses in these advanced practice roles are evidence-brokers (Gerrish et al. 2007), who conduct investigations in selected research and development topics, and evaluate and report on the application of research and development findings within practice (Skills for Health 2009).

Exploratory semi-structured interviews and focus group interviews were conducted by the action research co-facilitators (Bellman and Wiseman 2010) with representative participants at all levels of the organisation. Participants were: patient governors, executive and senior managers, nurses and midwives, medical and library colleagues. Semi-structured interviews were also conducted with senior academic and executive staff within partnership universities and the Strategic Health Authority. The Consultant co-researchers chose to conduct exploratory interviews in their specialist field of practice with executive and senior managers, clinical nurses and midwives, Allied Health Professionals, and medical colleagues. The key findings to emerge were:

- the continuing struggle: for nursing and midwifery staff to conduct small scale, practice-based, high impact research in a current culture that values large scale, externally funded medical research;
- the invisibility of nursing and midwifery research: that had been and was being conducted within the hospital;
- the lack of continuity of support: within the hospital for nursing and midwifery research and development;
- the need for academic input into clinical contexts: as a key support for staff.

This phase of the project contributed to a successful outcome: strategic support, including ring-fenced funding, for a centre for nurse- and midwife-led research and development in the hospital trust. A long term vision and adequate resources with sustained funding are now minimum requirements. To enable the development of practice-based research the following objectives are suggested:

- Create a sustainable hospital infrastructure, to include clinical academic systems, to support practice-based research and development and evidence-informed practice;
- Engage with key stakeholders, including service users, practitioners, managers and academic colleagues, in developing a practice-based research and development culture in the hospital trust;
- Support consultant nurses/advanced practitioners and academic colleagues in engaging practitioners in nursing research and evidence-informed practice in clinical settings.

Two examples of practice-based research and development projects undertaken with clinical and academic colleagues are: a dignity and respect UK hospital-wide project (Crow et al. 2009), and a Canadian action research project to reduce the barriers to the delivery of safe, compassionate, competent and ethical care in clinical settings (Storch et al. 2009).

Conclusion

This chapter has provided practical insights into engaging in clinical action research in diverse practice settings. Whether as a small-scale patient-centred project or a hospital-wide project, the methodology enables healthcare professionals, educators and researchers, patients and carers to research together to advance patient care. The clinical action researcher needs to create an open and supportive environment in which to build trust, explore caring values and ensure power is shared within the group. Whether a novice to the methodology or a more experienced researcher, successful engagement in this collaborative 'culture of enquiry' (Winter & Munn-Giddings 2001) enables the clinical action researcher and co-researchers to improve and advance patient care, dissipate workplace conflict, increase their understanding of the research process, advance their professional knowledge, and recognise opportunities for future practice and professional development. However, not all planned and well-intentioned projects succeed for many of the reasons identified within this chapter. An integrated clinical academic approach, together with research funding and management support, will enhance understanding of the need for clinical action research and increase its impact on contemporary healthcare practice and patient outcomes.

Further reading

International Practice Development Journal http://www.fons.org/library/journal.aspx

Street, A (1995) *Nursing Replay: Researching Nursing Culture Together*. Melbourne: Churchill Livingsdtone.

Walsgrove, H and Fulbrook, P (2005) Advancing the clinical perspective: A practice development project to develop the nurse practitioner in an Acute Hospital Trust. *Journal of Clinical Nursing*. 14: 444–455.

Useful websites

Academy of Nursing Midwifery & Health Visiting Research (UK): www.research academy.co.uk/. The Academy of Nursing, Midwifery and Health Visiting Research has been established as a collaborative enterprise by the Royal College of Nursing, CPHVA – UNITE and the Royal College of Midwives in partnership with The Council of Deans for Health, the Nurse Directors group of the Association of UK University Hospitals, the Association for Leaders in Nursing, the Queen's Nursing Institute, Mental Health Nurse Academics UK, the UK Clinical Research Facility Network and Nurses in Primary Care Research.

ALARA (Action Research & Action Learning Association): www.alara.net.au/public/home. To promote by all available means the scientific study, practice, research and teaching of Action Learning, Action Research and Process Management, and to bring together those of whatsoever professional discipline who are concerned with AL, AR and PM.

FoNS (The Foundation of Nursing Studies *Centre for Nursing Innovation.*): www.fons.org/. The aims of FoNS are to inspire and enable nurses to lead innovation and change in nursing and healthcare practice to improve patient care. Within the Centre for Nursing Innovation you can access action research resources and studies from:

- a library of information about leading and facilitating innovation and change;
- a Learning Zone containing useful tools and resources;
- a Common Room where you can interact with others;
- programmes of support, facilitation and funding.

Involve: www.involve.org.uk. Involve are public participation specialists; bringing institutions, communities and citizens together to accelerate innovation, understanding discussion and change. Involve makes a practical difference by delivering the highest quality public participation processes possible as well as undertaking rigorous research and policy analysis into what works.

MindTools.com: www.mindtools.com: Theoretical guidance and practical advice on conflict resolution.

Steinberg Collection of nursing research: www.rcn.org.uk/development/library_steinberg_collection_of_nursing_research. The RCN Steinberg Collection is a unique reference collection of over 1,000 UK doctoral theses from the 1950s to the present day and masters dissertations to the year 2000 completed by nurses and others on topics of relevance to nursing.

References

Archer A & Cameron D (2009) *Collaborative Leadership. How to succeed in an interconnected world.* London: Butterworth-Heinemann.

Argyris C and Schön D (1974) *Theory in practice: Increasing professional effectiveness*, San Francisco: Jossey-Bass.

Bate P (2000) Synthesizing Research and Practice: Using the Action Research Approach in Health Care Settings. *Social Policy and Administration*, 34(4), 478–493.

Bellman L (2003) Nurse-led Change & Development in Clinical Practice. Nursing Research Series. London: Wiley-Blackwell.

Bellman L Bywood C & Dale S (2003) Advancing working and learning through critical action research: creativity and constraints. *Nurse Education in Practice*, 3 (4): 186–194.

Bellman L & Corrigan P (2010) Using action research to develop a thoracic support nurse role to enhance quality of care. *Nursing Times*, June 8–14; 106 (22): 18–21.

Bellman L Webster J & Jeanes A (2011) Knowledge transfer and the integration of research, policy and practice for patient benefit. *Journal of Research in Nursing*, 16(3): 254–270.

Bonner A & Tolhurst G (2002) Insider outsider perspectives of participant observation. *Nurse Researcher*, 9(4), 7–19.

Bridges J & Meyer J (2007) Exploring the effectiveness of action research as a tool for organisational change in health care. *Journal of Research in Nursing*, 12 (4): 389–399.

Carlson C and Plonczynski D (2008) Has the BARRIERS scale changed nursing practice? An integrative review. *Journal of Advanced Nursing*, 63(4), 322–333.

Carr W and Kemmis S (1986) *Becoming Critical. Education, knowledge and action research.* Lewes: Falmer.

Coghlan D & Brannick T (2010) *Doing Action Research in Your Own Organization*. Sage: 3rd edition.

Coghlan D & Casey M (2001) Action research from the inside: issues and challenges in doing action research in your own hospital. *Journal of Advanced Nursing*, Vol. 35, Number 5, September 2001, pp. 674–682(9).

Cohen D Crabtree B (2006) 'Qualitative Research Guidelines Project.' Available on line at http://www.qualres.org/HomeCrab-3492.html. Accessed July 2010.

Crow J Smith L & Keenan I (2009) Sustainability in an action research project: 5 years of a Dignity and Respect action group in a hospital setting. *Journal of Research in Nursing*. (doi: 10.1177/1744987109352929).

Eccles C (2009) Effective delivery of evidence-informed practice. *Evidence & Policy*, 5 (2): 193–206.

Elliott J (1978) What is action research in schools? *Journal of Curriculum Studies*, vol. 10, pp. 355–357.

Elsey H & Lathlean J (2006) Using action research to stimulate organisational change within health services: experiences from two community-based studies. *Educational Action Research*, 14, (2), 171–186. (doi:10.1080/09650790600718019)

Gerrish K Guillaume L Kirshbaum M McDonnell A Nolan M Read S Tod A (2007) Empowering frontline staff to deliver evidence-based care: The contribution of nurses in advanced practice roles. Available online at www.shu.ac.uk/hsc/sp-kate-gerrish. Accessed July 2010.

Glasson J Chang E Chenoweth L Hancock K Hall T & Hill-Murray F (2006) Evaluation of a model of nursing care for older patients using participatory action research in an acute medical ward. *Journal of Clinical Nursing*. Volume 15, Issue 5, pages 588–598. (doi: 10.1111/j.1365-2702.2006.01371.x)

Hockley J (2006) Developing high quality end-of-life care in nursing homes an action research study. Unpublished PhD thesis, University of Edinburgh & Steinberg collection, RCN.

Kemmis S (2006) Participatory action research and the public sphere. *Educational Action Research* Vol. 14, No. 4, December 2006, pp. 459–476, (doi: 10.1080/09650790600975593)

La Pine M P (2008) The domain of nursing: developing practice through action research in the Intensive Care Unit. Unpublished Master of Nursing dissertation, Victoria University of Wellington.

Meyer J (1993) New paradigm research: the trials and tribulations of action research. *Journal of Advanced Nursing*, vol. 18, pp. 1066–1072.

Meyer J (1995) Stages in the process: a personal account. *Nurse Researcher*, Vol. 2, No. 3, pp. 24–37.

Meyer J Spilsbury K & Prieto J (1999) Comparison of findings from a single case in relation to those from a systematic review of action research. *Nurse Researcher*, 7 (2): 37–59.

MindTools.com (2010) Conflict Resolution: resolving conflict rationally and effectively. Available online at www.mindtools.com (Last accessed November 2010).

Munn-Giddings C McVicar A & Smith L (2008) Systematic review of the uptake and design of action research in published nursing research, 2000–2005. *Journal of Research in Nursing* 13: 465–477, (doi:10.1177/1744987108090297)

Munten G van den Bogaard J Cox K Garretsen H & Bongers I (2010) Implementation of evidence-based practice in nursing using action research: a review. *Worldviews on Evidence-Based Nursing*, 7(3): 135–57.

Porter S (1996) Qualitative Research In Cormack D F S (ed) *The Research Process in Nursing*, Blackwell Scientific Publications, 3rd edition.

Roth J Shani A B (Rami) & Leary M M (2007) Insider action research: Facing the challenges of new capability development within a biopharma company. *Action Research* vol. 5 no. 1 41–60. (doi: 10.1177/1476750307072875)

Schipper K Abma T A A van Zadelhoff E van de Griendt J Nierse C & Widdershoven, G A A (2010) What does it mean to be a patient research partner? An ethnodrama. *Qualitative Inquiry*, 16 (6):501–510.

Skills for Health (2009) Nationally Transferable Roles. Advanced Practitioner Roles. Available online at www.skills for health.org.uk. Accessed July 2010.

Spalding N J (2009) Improving practice through involvement in action research. *International Journal of Therapy and Rehabilitation*, vol 16 (3): 130–138.

Streubert Speziale H J & Carpenter D R (2007) *Qualitative Research in Nursing: Advancing the Humanistic Imperative*. London: Lippincott Williams & Wilkins.

Storch J Rodney P Pauly B Fulton TR Stevenson L Newton L Makaroff K S (2009) Enhancing ethical climates in nursing work environments. *Canadian Nurse*. 105(3): 20–5

Toulmin S & Gustavsen B (eds) (1996) *Beyond Theory: Changing Organizations Through Participation*. John Benjamins Publishing.

Walmsley J & Mannan H (2009) Parents as co-researchers: a participatory action research initiative involving parents of people with intellectual disabilities in Ireland. *British Journal of Learning Disabilities*. (doi: 10.1111/j.1468-3156.2009.00582.x)

Waterman H Tillen D Dickson R & de Koning K (2001) Action research: a systematic review and guidance for assessment. *Health Technology Assessment* 5, 23 (executive summary). Available online at www.ncchta.org/fullmono/mon523.pdf. Accessed June 2010.

Webb C (1989) Action research, philosophy, methodology – personal experience. *Journal of Advanced Nursing*, vol. 14, pp. 403–410.

Wicks P G & Reason P (2009) Initiating action research: Challenges and paradoxes of opening communicative space. *Action Research* (2009) 7(3): 243–263.

Williams A M Dawson S S & Kristjanson L J (2008) Translating theory into practice: Using Action Research to introduce a coordinated approach to emotional care. *Patient Education & Counseling* 73: 82–90.

Williamson G & Prosser S (2002) Illustrating the ethical dimensions of action research. *Nurse Researcher* 10(2): 39–49.

Wingfield K (2008) Strategic thinkers in the making. *Cancer Nursing Practice*, 7 (8): 10.

Winter R & Munn-Giddings (2001) *A Handbook for Action Research in Health & Social Care*. London: Routledge.

Woodward V Webb C & Prowse M (2007) The perceptions and experiences of nurses undertaking research in the clinical setting. *Journal of Research in Nursing*, vol 12 (3): 227–244.

SECTION 3

CONDUCTING ACTION RESEARCH IN CLINICAL PRACTICE

5

DEVELOPING ONE'S OWN PROFESSIONAL PRACTICE

Jonathan Webster

Chapter objectives

Clinical action research can form an integral part of developing one's own practice. This chapter describes the experiential learning and insight I gained as a Consultant Nurse and clinical action research facilitator. Whether a small-scale project or one that extends beyond one clinical area, this narrative of my journey is offered to enable you to:

- appreciate the systematic and rigorous approaches that I used;
- consider how I have highlighted that working collaboratively with others can be complex;
- reflect on the frequently challenging and constantly evolving 'real world' context in which clinical action research is carried out.

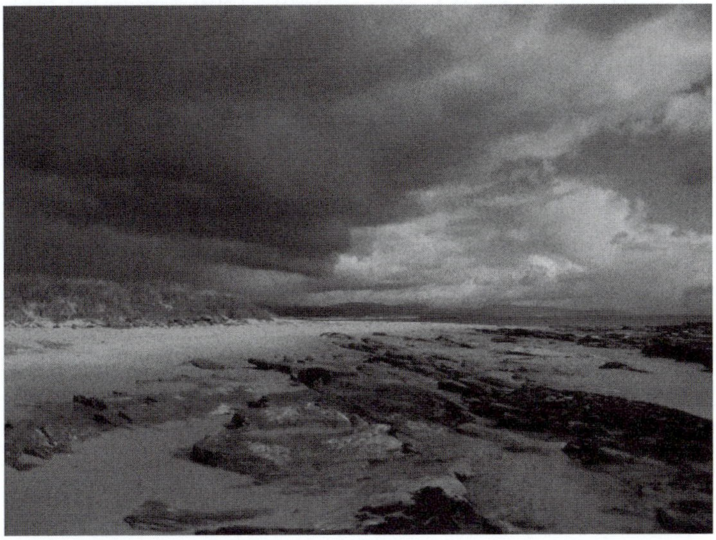

For the novice action researcher immersed in the complexity of clinical care, the narrative may also demystify some of the complex organisational cultures which can appear baffling and highly challenging. For the more experienced action researcher, although the challenges may remain, the experience and learning gained from leading and being part of previous action research studies can be highly valuable in helping to navigate and make sense of what and why something is happening, including issues that may have not been predicted. I wrote this poem to describe my journey:

> Waves beating against a sandy shore,
> The smell, sound and touch of the sea assault my senses,
> Invigorating, calming and yet frightening,
> I hear the waves talking, whispering words I can't hear but yet sense,
> I consider my journey along the sand, across sharp shells that make me step quicker,
> Soft sand that engulfs my feet and rock pools where I linger,
> Some of my footprints are visible, others are washed away,
> I look forward; I see where I want to go,
> I sense my inner strength and determination having got this far,
> Some of my footprints will remain, others will be washed away,
> But footprints will always be left in the soul.
> 'Footprints of an emancipatory practice development journey.'

Background to the action research study

In October 2001 I took up the post of Consultant Nurse for Older People within a District General Hospital (Webster 1999, 2007). The role was new to the Trust; the National Service Framework (NSF) for Older People (Department of Health 2001a) had just been published, a key expectation being that all general hospitals would have a nursing structure with clearly identified nurse leaders with responsibility for older people.

At that time, the post of the Consultant Nurse was a recent health service development, announced as a Government initiative in 1998. A commitment to establish the new role was outlined in the national strategy document *Making a Difference*, launched in July 1999 (Department of Health 1999) (Box 5.1). The first six months of the appointment was spent working in different clinical areas (within both the hospital and the community), identifying opportunities and challenges in older people's care, hearing older people's and their supporters' stories and the perceptions of staff about what did and didn't work well. Investment in this time was key as it enabled me to:

- build professional relationships with different stakeholders;
- understand the local agenda and priorities from a clinical practice perspective;
- identify where clinical expertise and energies should be directed as an agenda was emerging that was vast and unmanageable for one person alone.

Trying to understand how the Trust worked, the organisational and workplace cultures within the organisation and how 'things' happened was essential.

Box 5.1

Background to the Consultant Nurse post

This new 'super nurse' (BBC 1999) was expected to have a similar status to that of medical consultants and for the first time gave recognition that expert nurses would be enabled to remain at the bedside, delivering improved services for patients and in the context of gerontological practice 'truly modernising services for older people' (Sturdy 2004). Although these posts were broadly welcomed (Castledine 1999; Mellor 2001), some warned that they 'may divide the profession' (Scott 2000) and not achieve the goals intended due to the 'political manoeuvrings of others within the inter-professional team' (Jasper 2006). It was also recognised that the success of the role was dependent on its 'fit' within the organisation (Manley and Dewing 2002). At this time within the literature, there was a small amount of published research-based evaluation of these roles (Booth et al. 2006; Guest et al. 2004; Redfern 2006; Woodward et al. 2005). The majority of publications were, however, anecdotal reports or non-research-based discussion and narrative.

Four key elements of responsibility were defined for all Consultant Nurse posts by the National Health Service Executive (1999):

- Expert practice
- Professional leadership and consultancy
- Education and development
- Practice and service development linked to research and evaluation

Manley (1997) suggests that no matter how much practical and theoretical expertise an Advanced Practitioner/Consultant Nurse has, this on its own is of little value. Such posts must always be linked to their ultimate purpose of improving the quality of services to patients and their families. The Consultant Nurse does this by helping staff to see themselves as leaders and by facilitating a culture that values person-centred care.

A key corner stone to my role as a Consultant Nurse was 'Research and Development' and I was keen to incorporate this element into my post so that it was an integral part of what I did and not separate and disconnected from day-to-day working. Previously, Masters level study had enabled me to synthesise research and practice through practitioner-centred research (Webster 1999). I recognised the value and power of research that is generated from, is owned and clearly embedded in real-life clinical practice, the outcome being to inform and develop clinical care leading to change for patient benefit when needed.

Rationale for the study

The underpinning rationale for the study came from priorities I identified as a 'new' Consultant Nurse for Older People in the first six months. I had been given a 'blank sheet of paper' and while there were clear objectives I needed to deliver on within an agreed time span, I had been given the scope and authority to shape and craft the role to ensure that it met 'real' needs and priorities. These priorities were identified by working with teams in clinical practice both within and outside the Trust and by talking to and working with older people and their supporters. Balanced against this were key 'drivers' for change and modernisation such as the NSF for Older People (DOH 2001a) and a need to focus upon the 'essential' elements of care (DOH 2001b). At a time when there had been much policy activity based on reform and modernisation, in which the aim had been to improve health and healthcare for patients and communities (DOH 2000), policy needed to be seen as being a central part of underpinning service development and not in abstract or isolation.

More recent publications, such as *A new ambition for old age* (DOH 2006), were seen as reaffirming this through the three themes of 'Dignity in Care', 'Joined-Up Care' and 'Healthy Ageing'. A review of the progress in implementing the NSF for Older People, published by the Healthcare Commission (2006), highlighted that although there had been 'significant progress', there were 'further actions required' if it was to bring about 'real' changes in both the type of services and attitudes of staff working with older people.

Insight gained from talking with and listening to older people and their supporters, and observing and being part of practice, helped me to understand the priorities from a patient, professional and service delivery perspective. In identifying the priorities, I couldn't divorce my own values, beliefs and experiences of developing expert person-centred practice in the care of older people, based on past experiences and reflections both 'in' and 'on' action (Schön 1999) as these values, beliefs and experiences were key elements that informed my own thinking and actions. Individual people, different pieces of literature and academic study had also shaped my thinking and professional development.

Influences from practice – identifying a 'need' in practice

A recurrent theme that emerged from practice was how people were seen as they got older and healthcare professionals' understanding and perceptions of ageing. This was brought to the fore in different ways. Frequently I observed discussions between professionals that appeared to devalue the sense of who the older person was or phrases that potentially 'labelled' the person either intentionally or unintentionally. I observed that often discussions were about what the older person 'couldn't' or 'wouldn't' do; very little attention seemed to be paid to what they could do or indeed the person's desires and aspirations for the future. On occasions, such discussions were about the person's future, without consulting the person first and, importantly, ascertaining what they wanted or hoped for. At times I felt that the 'patient' (the older person) had become disconnected from their past and who they were – knowing the person, what was important to them and who they were was not always seen as being integral to providing holistic, therapeutic care (Box 5.2).

Box 5.2

I was working one morning with a Care Assistant on a busy, acute ward. One of the ladies we were looking after had suffered a stroke. I entered her room and observed her sitting next to her bed. There was a table in front of her and a glass of water. I said 'hello' and who I was. I received no response. The care assistant I was working with said, 'Don't worry, she never responds'.

As we started to make the lady's bed, the person I was working with started to talk to me about my role; it was as if the patient wasn't there. I asked, 'Does this lady ever wear make-up?' The person I was working with replied, 'I wouldn't have thought so.' I looked in her bedside locker and found a make-up bag. Immediately when I put it in front of the lady she became animated, she opened it and started applying foundation, lip stick and perfume. The care assistant I was working with was amazed. She said, 'I just never knew that she could do this'. We ensured that this information was included in the care plan and that it was handed over to oncoming staff so that this activity became central to nursing care.

I observed that frequently practitioners hadn't tried to find out about the person. At times I was told that this was due to the pressure of work and lack of perceived time. As an experienced nurse, however, I felt that in some cases the time that was available was not used effectively to engage with older people about what was important to them based on past life experiences, present needs and desires, and aspirations for the future. I also recognised that for some practitioners this was a 'safe' way to practise as it was easier to 'do the job' – it required little problem solving or critical reflection and reinforced traditional relationships based on power or 'I know what is best for you' rather than asking the person 'How can I help you?'. Taylor (1992) suggests that nurses and patients share a common humanity, a humanity so ordinary that it is often over-looked by attempts to professionalise nursing.

I witnessed on two different occasions two scenarios about how nurses worked with and cared for older people. The first of these scenarios is presented in Box 5.3.

Box 5.3

On one occasion I had arranged to work in a clinical area on an early shift. I arrived on the ward and was met by a Staff Nurse who asked me 'What are you going to do about all these old people who are blocking our beds?' Later during the shift I was asked to look after a man who had complex age-related needs. A different Staff Nurse stated 'He's been driving us mad as he is so demanding, let's see what you can do!' What became evident very quickly working with this man was that he was frightened about the situation in which he found himself. Before his acute, sudden illness he had led a very independent life. He had been in hospital for five weeks and during that time had spent two weeks in Intensive Care where he had received one-to-one attention. He was now in an open ward. He still required a high level of acute care interventions, however, through discussion as part of caring for him, what became obvious was that he felt that he had no future. It appeared that he had become disconnected from his past, who he was, and what was important to him, his life and his family.

During my time working with him for the shift I was able to find out more about him, based on what he was happy to disclose and share. As part of care, he had particular requirements and liked belongings and personal possessions to be placed in a certain way. I recognised that he wasn't 'being demanding' but was exerting control over something that he could focus on, as he had felt that he had lost control over so many other parts of his life. In reading the man's assessments and care plans, none of these elements was captured. Instead he had core care plans that were one-dimensional, that described universal tasks such as 'washing' and 'drain management'. Information that was needed to help those caring for him to see what was important to him and to understand him as a person was missing.

What this example highlighted to me was a need to help nurses see past the 'elderly patient' to an older person who has a past, present and future, and a need to focus on therapeutic care that is driven by the older person based on what they want, not on what the professional thinks, is important. Underpinning this is the ability to capture the attributes that represent our humanness (Webster and Whitlock 2003). Themes around how assessments were carried out with older people emerged as being important, as the process of assessment provides the 'building blocks' on which care is built. However, frequently assessment is based predominantly on direct physical observation and not on human observation that is seen by some as being 'inconsistent' and 'unreliable' (Stuart 2003). Barker (1997) further suggests that nurses have begun to realise that nursing assessment is not primarily concerned with the diagnosis of illness, rather the identification of a wide range of human needs that occur when a person experiences ill health.

Working with older people and their supporters and different teams helped me to identify the key emerging themes from practice; specifically, how nursing assessments were carried out with older people and the value placed on the process of assessment as part of a continuum or 'journey'. Integral to this was how older people were seen as 'elderly patients' who were 'ill' or 'unable to cope at home', people who had become 'disconnected' from who they were. I was told by some nurses that 'individualised nursing care' was practised and that 'we treat all patients as individuals'. However, based on observation and discussion, I was uncertain what this really meant (are the therapeutic nursing needs of every person the same?) and how was 'individuality' embedded in the workplace culture and reflected in day-to-day therapeutic working with older people? It seemed that finding out about the person, what was important to them and putting their desires and aspirations for the present and future at the centre of all activity needed to be more than 'caring' or 'empathy' based on an individual practitioner's own values and beliefs (this has been reported in part in Webster 2009).

Developing a research question – why action research?

Action research was chosen as the methodology of choice for the study as it enabled the research question ('To what extent has a programme of emancipatory practice development[1] enabled nurses working with older people to develop person-centred assessment within an acute hospital Trust?') to be explored. Within nursing, action research is focused on bridging the gap between theory, research and practice (Owen 1993), as its power lies in its use to develop greater collaboration and inclusiveness between practitioners and researchers (Manley and McCormack 2003; Reed 2005; Titchen and Binnie 1993; Titchen and Manley 2006) and critical reflective practice in which theory and practice are integrated, and in which theory may be generated from practice (Brown et al. 2003; Hart and Bond 1995; Meyer 1993; Roberts and Dick 2003,) through continuous spirals of planning, acting, observing and reflection (Atwal 2002; Grundy 1982). Action research was the most appropriate methodology to use in the study as its underpinning values of

[1]For the purpose of this chapter, 'practice development' is defined as '... a continuous process of improvement towards increased effectiveness in patient-centred care. This is brought about by helping healthcare teams to develop their knowledge and skills and to transform the culture and context of care. It is enabled and supported by facilitators committed to systematic, rigorous continuous process of emancipatory change that reflects the perspectives of service users' (Garbett and McCormack 2002: p 29), reflecting emancipatory or critical action research approaches (also see Chapters 1, 2, 3 and 4).

'closing the theory–practice gap' and its basis in 'real' practice to enable practice to change rather than 'learning' in isolation why certain activities occurred (Ferrance 2000). Furthermore, action research occurs 'in' practice rather than 'on' practice in which there is a clear focus on practitioner development, improvement and continuous learning (Dewar and Sharp 2006).

As identified in early chapters, a key attraction for practitioner researchers of action research is its practical, problem-solving nature, in which the researcher is able to work with study participants in a collaborative, inclusive, non-hierarchical and non-exploitative way (Bell 1993; Binnie and Titchen 1999; Coghlan and Casey 2001) and in which there is an opportunity to 'bring together' practitioners and researchers to enable greater partnerships, collaboration and inclusive ways of working (Reed 2005; Williams 2005). Furthermore, it is focused on closing the theory–practice gap, as its powers lie in its use to develop critical reflective practice and learning through interactive 'spiralling' cycles of identifying a problem, acting and evaluating (Argyris et al. 1985), in which theory and understanding are generated and gained from real-life practice (Hart and Bond 1995). Meyer (2001) further suggests that action research enables the practitioner to explore in detail practical concerns and ways of overcoming issues within the sometimes unpredictable and 'murky waters of reality' (for further understanding, see Chapter 3).

Challenges abound for the practitioner researcher who chooses action research due to the complexities of the 'real world' because of rapidly changing agendas at both national and local levels. As a Consultant Nurse working with older people, the pressures at times felt immense in supporting people while challenging their practice when around them the organisation in which they worked was undergoing change and development as part of the ongoing programmes of NHS modernisation, reform and fiscal scrutiny. Action research can be seen as being multidimensional and although the action researcher may have one key focus at the start of the study, other dimensions or elements may emerge which will lead to different pathways and avenues and at times may lead in totally different directions. Challenges and opportunities can also be seen in the relationships that the practitioner action researcher develops with both the teams and individuals with whom they are working.

A key challenge I found was that by the nature of critical inquiry and reflection, the issues that arose from practice appeared more complex than could be captured by a single 'spiral', as discussing a certain theme would lead in another direction for discussion and reflection-on-action. McNiff (1988: 37) concurs with this view and states: '... new issues would inevitably arise and have to be tackled separately, as new spirals of work.' Binnie and Titchen (1999) identified similar themes resulting from a four-year action research study of the development of 'patient-centred nursing' in Oxfordshire which aimed to 'unravel' the complex processes involved in change. Binnie and Titchen (1999) describe a 'tree of action spirals' that captures related themes within the context of action research. As the programme and study progressed, similar interrelated spirals emerged from the work which moved away from the study itself, however they remained focused upon developing practice with older people. These interrelated themes and spirals were very relevant and evident as part of the study as different practice development opportunities arose from the core piece of work with different clinical areas. Two of the clinical areas that took part in the programme subsequently asked me to work with them and their teams on a programme of 'Observations of Care'. I was asked to present at a team away day on person-centred assessment for one of the clinical areas. I became a clinical supervisor for two of the participants once the programme had formally finished and a video was made with two of the participating areas on person-centred practice which was used on the Trust Induction Programme and for training and education. As a Consultant Nurse, these pieces of work not only reflected the evolutionary development of a piece of action research, but the growth and development of my own role within a complex and rapidly changing health and social care system.

In the action research study I felt that my role was blurred as I wore many hats at different times:

- as a Consultant Nurse for Older People and Senior Nurse working within the Trust;
- as a practice developer;
- as a clinical action researcher who was investigating practice from a research perspective within my own organisation; and
- as a postgraduate student studying for a PhD.

On many occasions these roles became blurred. A key danger was that objectivity was potentially replaced by subjectivity as a result of the day-to-day challenges associated with working in the 'context' of my own organisation, which at times felt immensely 'complex'. Personal reflection (using a reflective journal) along with formal supervision (clinical and research) became an essential part of my own development and support during this time, as it helped me maintain the degree of objectivity and self-awareness that I felt was needed. It would have been easy to have become 'lost' in the unpredictable and frequently challenging and complex world of both clinical practice and organisational priorities.

Structure

The study was made up of three action research cycles and ran in total for two and a half years (each cycle lasted for approximately nine months).

Within each cycle there were five distinct phases (see Box 5.4). Before the programme started, I sought agreement from both the Director of Nursing and Head of Practice Development to take forward this programme of work. Their support and buy-in was key, not only in supporting me as a Consultant Nurse, but also in acting as both a 'shield' if needed and advocates for the programme.

Box 5.4

Phase 1

I met with the Ward Sister to discuss the content and structure of the programme of practice development. At this stage the Ward Sister was asked to identify those staff they would like to take part in the programme and the commitment needed to release them from practice. Engaging with the Ward Sister at this early stage ensured that a commitment to support the programme of practice development was made explicit from the outset and that 'ownership' sat with the Ward Sister. It was also important at this stage to gauge the level of ongoing support that team members would have within the context of developing practice and the formal methods and structures for dissemination and sharing information across the team.

To gain a greater understanding of clinical practice with older people within the areas taking part, I worked alongside the nursing team in the clinical setting. This not only supported a greater understanding of real practice and what happened on a 'day-to-day' basis, but also helped me to observe how the team worked with and engaged older people as part of clinical practice, and how they communicated and worked with each other and the broader multi-professional team. Snow (2002) asserts that participant observation can be the most accurate way of measuring the 'organisational climate' and the reality of what happens in the 'real world' and an understanding of the culture as a 'living entity' (Wilson et al. 2005). This period of working together formed the foundation of a professional relationship between me and the clinical areas taking part, both as part of the study in which participants were seen as being co-researchers in action research and in relation to the practice development and expert practice components of the Consultant Nurse role.

Phase 2

All nurses working within the clinical areas taking part were asked to complete a values clarification (see Chapter 6) to help identify where they were in their thinking and understanding of the process of assessment with older people and the values and beliefs underpinning their practice. This helped to identify the espoused values and beliefs of staff related to the importance they placed on the process of assessment with older people and to gain an understanding of the workplace characteristics.

Based on previous experience, I recognised that frequently espoused values, i.e. what people believe to be 'right', was not always reflected in the 'reality' of day-to-day clinical practice. Therefore observations from Phase 1 and these data collected from Phase 2 was key to understanding the culture and real-life context of clinical care underpinning practice with older people in the areas taking part.

Phase 3

Once identified by the Ward Sister, the participants were invited to attend a briefing meeting to identify the frequency and time for the practice development sessions. The day and time that the group met was decided by the group, as it was recognised that as part of 'owning' the programme, it needed to fit in with clinical commitments such as shift patterns, ward meal times and nursing handover. At this stage a briefing letter was given to all participants. This was also copied to their manager to reaffirm the commitment, i.e. release from practice, to participate in the programme. After the briefing meeting, it was agreed that each of the practice development sessions would occur once every two weeks and would last for two hours. These were divided into two parts:

- exploring the theory underpinning the principles of assessment and person-centred practice with older person;
- reflecting on personal learning based on activities with specific themes.

This part of the programme lasted for about 20 weeks. A focus of action research involving groups is that activities will need to be coordinated and helped either by an individual or a small group of researchers (Grundy 1982). Within this context, I took on this role, in which I not only acted as a facilitator but became a resource in which the group could draw on (see Chapter 6). Accompanying each session were briefing notes on the area covered for that week with supporting literature and related published research. Supporting those taking part in both the programme and the study to enable them to explore their practice with older people was key to help develop learning and greater insight and understanding into their practice.

A key focus of action research is to develop co-investigative partnerships with those who, under a traditional research paradigm, may be viewed as the 'subjects' for investigation. Dewar and Sharp (2006) suggest that such approaches, in which participants are seen as co-researchers, can lead to 'communities of inquiry' in which participants are engaged in questioning their own attitudes, actions and behaviours. As this phase progressed, the theme became very evident as participants openly questioned and reflected upon both their own practice with older people and more broadly how the teams they were part of worked with older people.

At this stage of the study, written consent was not sought from participants (see below) as it formed part of the programme of practice development that I was working on with their clinical area. However, participants were aware that I would be using field notes as part of this phase which they verbally agreed to during the first session. Meyer et al. (2003) identify that action research can raise ethical issues related to confidentiality and consent as frequently observations can be recorded as a result of informal conversations with a variety of different people. For this reason, I needed to be clear and transparent throughout about my aims and intentions. I also needed to use my professional judgement in deciding what it was appropriate to record.

Phase 4

Before the first evaluation, written consent was sought from the participants (see Chapter 7). All participants had the option not to take part in the evaluation. Semi-structured interviews were completed with participants to identify how the process of learning (both taught and reflective) had influenced their thinking and practice

(Continued)

(Continued)

with older people. As part of this phase, the participants were also asked to draw a picture to describe their views of the programme. This acted not only as an 'ice breaker', but also provided a focus for discussion as those taking part were asked to describe the picture. This level of creativity felt appropriate for the evaluation as a key intention of the programme of practice development was focused on developing creativity in both professional practice with older people and thinking. Freshwater (2004) identifies that, through creativity, greater emotional intelligence can occur, which provides an opportunity to learn both about oneself and the way in which we relate to patients and colleagues. From a research perspective, Higgs and Titchen (2001) identify that tensions can occur in professional practice and research and between rational, intuitive and creative thinking and between art, craft and science. They argue that by making sense and valuing these different elements that underpin personal knowledge, an attempt can be made to 'bridge' the theory–practice gap. The use of art as part of this phase focused on enabling creative thinking, in which participants were free to express their views about the programme.

Phase 5

After three months each of the study participants were re-interviewed. The aim of this phase was to identify how or if they had used what they had learnt from the programme to influence the development of person-centred assessment with older people within their clinical areas and to identify the key challenges that they may have faced.

Developing one's own practice

Structured reflection through writing and clinical supervision played a key role in underpinning each of the three main action research cycles and as such enabled me to make sense of what was occurring during each stage of evolutionary development. Throughout the duration of the programme, I recognised that I wore different 'hats' at different stages. My primary role was that of a Consultant Nurse, however this also blended with being a PhD student, along with that of an action researcher and practice developer. Reflection helped me make sense of what I was doing and when, I was also able to recognise that in helping others to develop their practice through an action research emancipatory approach, I was using facilitation skills centred upon 'enabling others' rather than 'doing for others' (Loftus-Hills and Harvey 2000; see also Chapter 6).

Rolfe et al. (2001) argue that a key purpose of action research is to enable self-reflection in the practitioner, therefore discovering unrecognised shortcomings leading to improvements in practice. The interpretations of meanings are therefore contextual to the time and place. **Reflexivity** is a key component within the critical sciences where it is used to ensure that the area being examined is as far as is possible critically appraised. Rolfe et al. (2001) further suggest the important component of reflexive action research as it 'addresses' the reality of practice in both teaching and nursing, thereby bringing theory and practice closer together. In describing the synthesis of reflection and action, Wheeler and Chinn (1984) refer to this as 'praxis research', which they define as being 'thoughtful reflection' and 'action' that occur in synchrony with each other (see Chapter 1). Meyer (2001) further suggests that there has been a gradual change in thinking related to action research, which has moved away from **positivist** and interpretive notions of science to the more 'modern' understanding of action research in which there is an emphasis on practitioners as researchers and the importance of self-reflection in the development of a critical science through the empowerment of practitioners.

The four stages of development within the action research cycle (Lewin 1948), along with the refined three stages as described by Kemmis and McTaggart (1988) (both referred to in Chapter 1), provided a systematic approach to developing change and innovation within the social world, which leads to action followed by a period of reflection. However, it could be argued that for the expert practitioner (Benner 1984) involved with making sense of highly complex situations that need immediate action while attempting to gain a greater understanding of the context of the situation, it is far less easy to compartmentalise reflection into a 'subset' of professional practice as it forms an integral part of expert practice (Fowler 2006; O'Callaghan 2005; Woodall 2000) and an automatic, intuitive part of how the expert practitioner functions due to the synthesis and 'blending' of different types of knowledge, including experiential and theoretical knowledge.

While I recognised that my reflections were time-, place- and context-specific, my broader observations captured in my field notes and records enabled me to take a broader view of both the action research study and programme of practice development. They contributed, along with my reflections and formal evaluations within each cycle and the subsequent phases described in Box 5.4,) to the recurrent themes that emerged.

Emerging themes and learning from Cycle One

I recognised that as this cycle had progressed, taking forward the programme was going to be challenging as working with staff, in particular during Phase 3 (see Box 5.4) was going to require great flexibility, creativity and commitment due to the day-to-day demands on their time. Although I had achieved buy-in from the Ward Sisters, I sensed that the programme was potentially perceived as yet another commitment (although valued) that had to compete with the other demands that their clinical areas were facing. Early in this first cycle, I had questioned if the programme should continue since only one participant remained (Anne). However, although not ideal, I recognised the impact that the programme had made on her practice and the subsequent leadership she was providing for her team. I felt that, although initially uncertain, the method of delivery was appropriate and I observed how the reflective exercises helped link the themes for exploration into practice. The participant had used the reflective exercises to gain both a greater insight into and understanding of her practice with older people.

Working so closely with the one participant in cycle one, I gained a far greater insight and understanding of the real-life issues and complexities associated with developing practice with older people within an integrated healthcare system in which older persons' care was not always seen as being a specialist area of practice compared with single pathology specialities. Although on her ward the majority of patients were older people with complex multiple pathologies, the nursing and therapy team saw their identity as being a single pathology speciality. Themes had emerged through working with Anne, such as how the programme had 'liberated her practice' and that perceived barriers (which were subsequently not barriers at all) had previously stopped her working in a person-centred way. During the programme working with Anne, and more broadly with members of the nursing team, I sensed that her team was very keen to develop practice and were ready to describe changes in how they worked that kept the older person central to care. However, on occasions they appeared restrained due to systems, processes and ways of working that were in place, such as core assessments and care plans that fitted older people's needs into universal 'boxes'.

Through sharing, exploring and learning with Anne, and more broadly her team, I had learnt more about myself in how I was developing and enhancing my facilitation skills. I also recognised that through an emancipatory action research approach I was able to explore practice with older people from within. I was enabling Anne to critically reflect upon how she and her team worked with and cared for older people. However, I recognised that at this time this also led to challenges for me since it would have become easy to have become immersed in the workings of the team as I was constantly balancing being both an 'insider' and 'outsider'. Both clinical and research supervision proved invaluable early on. It enabled me to maintain a distance when needed but also to be able to step back into practice, therefore feeling able to move backwards and forwards along a continuum that joined the 'insider' and 'outsider' role (for further discussion of 'facilitation', see Chapter 6).

Emerging themes and learning from Cycle Two

I recognised that the participants were very committed to the programme and frequently would attend on their days off. I was less clear, however, whether they saw themselves as co-researchers, where we were all on the same journey. Although I had emphasised at the start of the programme the need to communicate with colleagues, I was uncertain as to how this happened, and although I had maintained links with the Ward Sisters at different times and had offered to give feedback on team away days or team meetings, I was unclear as to how this work was being owned by the teams and their leaders as a whole. At times I felt as if the programme sat in a 'bubble' on its own and although the participants were making the links to practice and how they worked with older people through the reflective exercises, there appeared to be little overall integration. Similarly, the concept of person-centred assessment was potentially perceived as being too challenging, as traditional ways of carrying out assessments were well established, accepted and liked, and they didn't necessarily challenge the traditional status quo.

This cycle evoked in me many mixed emotions. At times I had felt despairing of the constant, unrelenting challenges I faced in progressing the programme while developing my role. This, coupled with the need to reschedule sessions as participants were unable to be released from practice, people withdrawing in Phase 3 and having two remaining participants to interview in Phase 5, made me question at times the context in which an emancipatory action research approach could enable change and development when there appeared to be such continued 'turbulence'. Similarly, while the approach was enabling me to gain a real understanding through systematic, evolutionary spirals of development, at times I was unclear whether I felt 'comfortable' with what I was discovering, and the level of insight and understanding I was gaining because the realities of practice felt at 'odds' with what I believed (as a person) was important for older persons' care. At other times during this cycle I had been ecstatic at the enthused, creative exploration of practice with older people by committed participants through the use of narrative, in which there was a clear application of the learning from the programme. This learning was demonstrated in how they worked with older people, together with the observation that the programme was facilitating participants to develop person-centred ways of working (see Chapter 6).

I started to identify that for some participants, exploring person-centredness within the context of assessment may have been too complex, as they were still exploring and making sense of, within their own practice, ways of working that kept the older person and their supporters central to care. And although the process of assessment is key to systematic care planning and ongoing evaluation, at times it appeared to be a 'piece of paper' rather than the foundations on which care is planned. I also recognised that some ways of working were firmly entrenched in both the unspoken subcultures of the teams taking part and the culture of the organisation. Half way through Cycle Two, I spoke with a Senior Nurse of one of the participating areas as I wanted to offer my support for a change in practice that she was attempting to bring about. Her response was, 'I thought you were going to tell me off!' Initially I was very surprised at this. However, it reaffirmed to me at that time that the unseen workplace culture was not always supportive of changing practice for those who were trying to bring about positive changes to the patients' experience of care. I also become increasingly aware during this cycle of the key importance of understanding the characteristics of clinical leadership and how the qualities attributed to such leaders are transferred into work-based clinical cultures.

During this cycle, initially I had been baffled by the contradictions I had experienced. At times during Phase 1 I had observed practice that was routinised and task-centred. However, the values espoused by individuals who had completed the values clarification in Phase 2 expressed the opposite. This highlighted that although practitioners espoused a belief in care that was focused on the needs of the person, at times these values and beliefs were not reflected in day-to-day practice with older people. During this cycle, one participant identified to me that although she understood the importance of person-centred assessment, the culture of practice within the team enforced a non-person-centred way of working. Having modified the values clarification that was originally used in Cycle One during Cycle Two, the adapted tool now appeared more sensitive and helped identify these contradictions. I also recognised the importance of using multi-method approaches, i.e. to gain an understanding of practice, as potentially a single-method approach would not have captured the complexity underpinning practice with older people.

Similar themes were emerging across both action research cycles, such as the place of culture and leadership in practice along with the power of tradition and ritual. I also observed that the needs of people as they got older were frequently seen as being secondary compared to the primary acute pathology. This, in my view, highlighted the importance of ensuring that staff were both supported and enabled to develop sustainable, evidence-based skills and knowledge in the care of older people and that the workplace culture underpinning practice with older people needed to enable this to occur.

I decided that the approach taken to Cycle Three would mirror that of Cycle Two with no changes being made to the study along with the programme of practice development. However, I recognised that, as with this cycle, great flexibility would be needed to work with the participating areas and that although I would be using the same approach, new themes and needs may emerge that would require creative thinking and systematic problem solving, underpinned by critical reflection as part of the action research cycle.

Emerging themes and learning from Cycle Three

Similar themes emerged from this cycle which had resonance with the preceding two action research cycles. I had found working through this cycle increasingly challenging, primarily due to my own personal growth through Cycles One and Two and my personal feelings of frustration that although I could enable the development of person-centred assessment with older people so far, I had no direct influence in making it a reality within the areas I had been working because I had no direct operational influence.

Similarly, to me (throughout the whole study), participants of this cycle had clearly been on a journey and I noticed a change in how some of them approached working with and caring for older people. Over the 24 weeks in which we met, I also noticed a change in their level of engagement and commitment to taking the work forward. However, balanced against this were the challenges they faced on a daily basis related to clinical dependency, staffing and the general operational management of their clinical areas.

Recurrent themes that emerged from this cycle included the power of culture (workplace and organisational) within practice, in which the culture sets the scene as to how practitioners behave and work with older people. The place of transformational leadership was also identified as being key in challenging ways of working that were based on tradition and history in which care was mechanical, not critically reflective and non-person-centred. For some of the participants, the ability to critically reflect (in a non-superficial manner) in practice appeared too challenging. A reason was that at their level of practice, this degree of reflection 'in' and 'on' action may have appeared too daunting as it was not the cultural 'norm' at that stage in time (recognising that both areas had two new clinical leaders) within their clinical settings to reflect and gain greater insight and understanding from within practice.

At times participants appeared to feel powerless in challenging the use of core documentation that did not reflect the needs of older people, and although they recognised this on many occasions, they openly identified that it was 'one step too far' to try to change what other practitioners felt safe and comfortable with.

As with my reflections at the end of Cycle Two, I increasingly felt that the programme sat within a 'bubble' on its own and that emancipatory action research to enable practice to develop appeared to be at odds with others (albeit a minority) who preferred more technical approachs to training, learning and practice development. This was also reflected in facilitation styles, where I was focusing upon enabling others through 'seeking to explore and release the inherent potential of individuals' (Rycroft-Malone et al. 2004) compared to a practical and task-driven focus centred upon achieving specific tasks.

Having completed this Third Cycle, I was uncertain where the formal programme of developing person-centred assessment with older people would lead. I was sensing a tension between emancipatory and technical approaches to developing practice with older people because for some (not all) emancipatory action research appeared too challenging compared to more traditional, didactic technical approaches to developing both practice and practitioners. However, emancipatory action research helped me to make sense of what was happening both at a micro and macro level. I felt that I had been able to get 'under the skin' of practice and therefore make sense of and understand the complex interactions that were occurring.

Summary

The programme of practice development described encompassed an emancipatory/critical action research approach (within a framework of emancipatory practice development) which charted a journey of personal development not only for me as a Consultant Nurse/action researcher/practice developer, but also for those practitioners who took part in the journey with me. In developing my own practice, a number of themes emerged from the action research study (see Box 5.5). These have influenced future work with teams that have focused upon developing person-centred practice with older people. The outcome and evaluation of Cycle One, Cycle Two and Cycle Three reflected the development and evaluation of a strategy and modification testing of the programme of practice development within different clinical settings/environments, a key influencing element being the relationship between the researcher and study participants as co-researchers.

Box 5.5

- The importance of understanding the context of care.
- The importance and place of transformational leadership.
- Understanding and being able to work within the organisational imperatives.

- Understanding of 'role' that the facilitator takes within an emancipatory/critical action research approach and the ability to be able to move between different roles when needed.
- Understanding and influence of the culture (workplace and organisational) both at a micro and macro level and the subsequent influence on outcomes.

References

Argyris, C, Putnam, R and Smith, D (1985) *Action science*. San Francisco, CA: Jossey-Bass.

Atwal, A (2002) Getting the evidence into practice: The challenges and successes of action research. *British Journal of Occupational Therapy* 65(7): 335–341.

Barker, P (1997) *Assessment in psychiatric and mental health nursing: In search of the whole person*. Cheltenham: Stanley Thornes.

BBC (1999) 'Super nurses' arrive. Available online at: http://news.bbc.co.uk/1/hi/health/389998.stm (last accessed 1/7/ 2010).

Bell, J (1993) *Doing your research project*. Buckingham: Open University Press.

Benner, P (1984) *From novice to expert: Excellence and power in clinical nursing practice*. Menlo Park, CA: Addison-Wesley.

Binnie, A and Titchen, A (1999) *Freedom to practice: The development of patient-centred nursing*. Oxford: Butterworth Heinemann.

Booth, J, Hutchinson, C, Beech, C and Robertson, K (2006) New nursing roles: The experience of Scotland's consultant nurse/midwives. *Journal of Nursing Management* 14: 83–89.

Brown, D, Bammer, G, Batliwala, S and Kunreuther, F (2003) Framing practice-research engagement for democratizing knowledge. *Action Research* 1(1): 81–102.

Castledine, G (1999) Nurse consultants herald new era for clinical nursing. *British Journal of Nursing* 8(18): 1258.

Coghlan, D and Casey, M (2001) Action research from the inside: Issues and challenges in doing action research in your own hospital. *Journal of Advanced Nursing* 35(5): 674–682.

Department of Health (2009) Making a difference: Strengthening the nursing, midwifery and health visiting contribution to health and healthcare. http://www.dh.gov.uk/prod_consum_dh/groups/dh_digitalassets/@dh/@en/documents/digitalasset/dh_4074704.pdf (last accessed 14th July 2011).

Department of Health (2000) The NHS Plan, London: Stationary Office.

Department of Health (2001a) *The national service framework for older people*. London: The Stationery Office.

Department of Health (2001b) *The essence of care: Patient focused benchmarking for healthcare practitioners* (first version). London: The Stationery Office.

Department of Health (2006) *A new ambition for old age: Next steps in implementing the national service framework for older people*. London: The Stationery Office.

Dewar, B and Sharp, C (2006) Using evidence: How action learning can support individual and organisational learning through action research. *Educational Action Research* 14(2): 219–237.

Elliott, J (1981) *Action research: A framework for self evaluation in schools*. Working Paper No. 1, Teacher–pupil interaction and the quality of learning, London schools. Mimeo. Cambridge: Cambridge Institute of Education.

Ferrence, E (2000) *Themes in education: Action research*. North and Islands Regional Education Laboratory at Brown University, Providence, RI.

Fowler, J (2006) The importance of reflective practice for nurse prescribers. *Nurse-Prescribing* 4(3): 103–106.

Freshwater, D (2004) Emotional intelligence: Developing emotionally literate training in mental health. *Mental Health Practice* 8(4): 12–15.

Garbett, R and McCormack, B (2002) A concept analysis of practice development. *Nursing Times Research* 7(2): 87–100.

Grundy, S (1982) Three modes of action research.*Curriculum Perspectives* 2(3): 23–34.

Guest, D, Peccei, R, Rosenthal, P, Redfern, S, Wilson-Barnett, J, Dewe, P, Coster, S, Evans, A and Sudbury, A (2004) *An evaluation of the impact of nurse, midwife and health visitor consultants*. Report to the Department of Health. Available at: www.umds.ac.uk/depsta/pse/mancen/research/FINAL_Nurse_Consultants_Report_2005.pdf (last accessed 1/7/2010).

Hart, E and Bond, M (1995) *Action research for health and social care*. Buckingham: Open University Press.

Healthcare Commission (2006) *Living well in later life: A review of the progress against the national service framework for older people*. London: Healthcare Commission.

Higgs, J and Titchen, A (2001) *Professional practice in health, education and the creative arts*. Oxford: Blackwell Science.

Jasper, M (2006) Editorial. Consultant nurses and midwives – are you making a difference? *Journal of Nursing Management* 14: 81–82.

Kemmis, S and McTaggart, R (1988) *The action research planner*. Geelong, Vic.: Deacon University Press.

Lewin, G (1948) *Resolving social conflicts: Selected papers on group dynamics by Kurt Lewin*. New York: Harper and Brothers.

Loftus-Hills, A and Harvey, G (2000) *A review of the role of the facilitator in changing professional healthcare practice*. Oxford: RCN Institute.

Manley, K (1997) A conceptual framework for advanced practice: An action research project operationalizing an advanced practitioner/consultant nurse role. *Journal of Clinical Nursing* 6: 179–190.

Manley, K and Dewing, J (2002) The consultant nurse role. *NHS Journal for Healthcare Professionals*, May: 8–9.

Manley, K and McCormack, B (2003) Research approach and methodology. In K Manley, S Hardy, A Titchen, R Garbett and B McCormack (eds), [2005,] *Changing patients' worlds through nursing practice expertise*. Oxford: RCN Institute.

McCormack, B, Manley, K and Garbett, R (2004) *Practice development in nursing*. Oxford: Blackwell.

McNiff, J (1988) *Action research: Principles and practice*. London: Macmillan Education.

Mellor, I (2001) Walking with lions. *Community Practitioner* 74(4): 135.

Meyer, J (1993) Lay participation in care: A challenge for multidisciplinary teamwork. *Journal of Interprofessional Care* 7(1): 57–66.

Meyer, J (2001) Lay participation in care in a hospital setting. Nursing Praxis: Portsmouth, England: International.

Meyer, J, Johnson, B, Proctor, S, Bryar, R and Rozmovits, L (2003) Practitioner research: Exploring issues in relation to research capacity building. *Nursing Times Research* 8(6): 407–417.

National Health Service Executive (1999) *Nurse, midwife and health visitor consultants: Establishing posts and making appointments*. London: National Health Service Executive.

O'Callaghan, N (2005) The use of expert practice to explore reflection. *Nursing Standard* 19(39): 41–47.

Owen, S (1993) Identifying a role for the nurse teacher in the clinical area. *Journal of Advanced Nursing* 18: 816–825.

Redfern, S (2006) Examining the effectiveness of the nurse consultant role. *Nursing Times* 102(4): 23–24.

Reed, J (2005) Using action research in nursing practice with older people: Democratising knowledge. *Journal of Clinical Nursing* 14(5): 594–600.

Roberts, C and Dick, B (2003) Emancipatory design choices for action research practitioners. *Journal of Community and Applied Psychology* 13: 486–495.

Rolfe, G, Freshwater, D and Jasper, M (2001) Critical reflection for nursing and the helping professions. New York: Palgrave.

Rycroft-Malone, J, Seers, K, Titchen, A, Harvey, G, Kitson, A and McCormack, B (2004) What counts as evidence in evidence-based practice? *Journal of Advanced Nursing* 47(1): 81–90.

Schön, D (1999) *The reflective practitioner: How professionals think in action*. Aldershot: Avebury.

Scott, H (2000) Consultant nurse role may divide the profession. *British Journal of Nursing* 9(3): 128.

Snow, J (2002) Enhancing work climate to improve performance and retain valued employees. *Journal of Nursing Administration* 32: 393–397.

Stuart, C (2003) *Assessment, supervision and support in clinical practice*. London: Churchill Livingstone.

Sturdy, D (2004) Consultant nurses: Changing the future. *Age and Ageing* 33: 327–328.

Taylor, B (1992) From helper to human: A reconceptualization of the nurse as a person. *Journal of Advanced Nursing* 17: 1042–1049.

Titchen, A and Binnie, A (1993) Research partnerships: Collaborative action research in nursing. *Journal of Advanced Nursing* 18: 858–865.

Titchen, Aand Manley, K (2006) Spiralling towards transformational action research: Philosophical and practice journeys. *Educational Action Research* 14(3): 333–356.

Webster, J (1999) Practitioner-centred research: An evaluation of the implementation of the bedside hand-over. *Journal of Advanced Nursing* 30(6): 1375–1382.

Webster, J (2007) Person-centred assessment with older people: An action research study to explore registered nurses' understanding of person-centred assessment within a framework of emancipatory practice development. PhD thesis, University of Portsmouth, UK.

Webster, J (2009) Expertise in practice: Older people. In S Hardy, A Titchen, B McCormack and K Manley (eds), *Revealing nursing expertise through practitioner enquiry*. Oxford: Wiley-Blackwell.

Webster, J and Whitlock, M (2003) Patient or person? *Nursing Older People* 15(5): 38.

Wheeler, C and Chinn, P (1984) *Peace and power: A handbook of feminist process*. Buffalo, NY: Margaret Daughters.

Whyte, WF (ed.) (1991) *Participatory action research*. Newbury Park, CA: Sage.

Williams, T (2005) Work-based learning: A leadership development example from an action research study of shared governance implementation. *Journal of Nursing Management* 13(6): 490–499.

Wilson, V, McCormack, B and Ives, G (2005) Understanding the workplace culture of a special care nursery. *Journal of Advanced Nursing* 50(1): 27–38.

Woodall, T (2000) Clinical expertise: A realistic entity or a phenomenological fantasy? *Journal of Neonatal Nursing* 6(1): 21–25.

Woodward, V, Webb, C and Prowse, M (2005) Nurse consultants: Their characteristics and achievements. *Journal of Clinical Nursing* 14: 845–854.

6

COLLABORATIVE WORKING IN CLINICAL SETTINGS

Loretta Bellman and Jonathan Webster

In contemporary action research the emphasis is on researchers and practitioners working collaboratively, with a special focus on awareness-raising and empowerment (Kennedy 2001). There is an assumption that healthcare professionals collaborate to provide and enable quality healthcare. While the desire to collaborate is laudable and a key driving force for change, this may often be the exception rather than the rule. Establishing effective collaboration is fundamental in an action research project. Yet, some studies claiming to use action research methods have failed to demonstrate true collaborative intent (Hockley 2006).

Facilitation is the key to enable effective intra-professional, multi-professional and user/carer collaboration in an action research project. The role of facilitator arises directly from the action research principle of collaboration (Winter and Munn-Giddings 2001).

Chapter objectives

The focus of this chapter is to consider how the action researcher, as both autonomous practitioner and team member, facilitates collaboration in clinical settings both for patient benefit and professional knowledge development. The objectives of the chapter are to:

- explore collaboration and facilitation in clinical action research projects;
- consider the strengths and challenges of facilitation by drawing from examples from clinical practice;
- emphasise the need for greater clinical academic collaboration *and* facilitation.

In a climate constantly demanding efficiency, cost-effectiveness and quality improvement professional collaboration warrants re-examination (Lindeke and Sieckert 2005). A key goal in healthcare is to improve effectiveness, through understanding and systematic change, leading to improved outcomes for patients. The strength of action research lies in the opportunity for team learning and change which is grounded in the context of services and pursued through collaboration (Hall 2006).

Collaboration and teamwork

Understanding the concepts of collaboration and teamwork are fundamental to engaging in action research. Teamwork and collaboration are often used synonymously (Thomas et al. 2003) and overlap in practice (see Box 6.1). The concept of collaboration encompasses the team approach but also requires the attribute of building a consensus – to enable team agreement and commitment to action.

Box 6.1

Attributes of a concept analysis of collaboration and teamwork

Collaboration (Henneman et al. 1995)	**Teamwork** (Xyrichis and Ream 2008)
1 Joint venture	1 Concerted effort
2 Co-operative endeavour	2 Interdependent collaboration
3 Willing participation	3 Shared decision-making
4 Shared planning and decision-making	
5 Team approach	
6 Contribution of expertise	
7 Shared responsibility	
8 Non-hierarchical relationships	
9 Power is shared and is based on knowledge and expertise rather than role or title	

Reaching a consensus is also required.

The conceptualisation of collaboration proposed by Gardner (2005) recognises that the concept is both a process (a series of events) and an outcome (a synthesis of different perspectives):

> Collaboration is both a process and an outcome in which shared interest or conflict that cannot be addressed by any single individual is addressed by key stakeholders. A key stakeholder is any party directly influenced by the actions others take to solve

> a complex problem. The collaborative process involves a synthesis of different perspectives to better understand complex problems. A collaborative outcome is the development of integrative solutions that go beyond an individual vision to a productive resolution that could not be accomplished by any single person or organization.

Contemporary support for an integrated approach to process and outcomes is evident in regard to inter-agency collaboration in health and social care research (Glasby and Dickinson 2008). The authors are critical of current approaches to research/evaluation and policy and practice that:

- fail to fully involve people who use services and frontline staff;
- only consider a narrow range of quantitative indicators, rather than adopting a broader approach that combines qualitative and quantitative research with consideration of the expertise of frontline practitioners and the lived experience of people who use the services;
- do not specifically identify the impact of collaboration;
- see collaboration as an end in itself rather than a means to an end.

• • • REFLECTIVE ACTIVITY 6.1 • • •

Consider the attributes of teamwork and collaboration in Box 6.1. How do they 'fit' within your uni-professional, multi-professional and patient-centred ways of working?

Engaging in a clinical action research project is a learning process which requires the systematic documentation of how collaboration with colleagues, patients, carers and other key stakeholders is initiated and sustained, together with the patient-centred changes that result. The contextual requirements for collaboration have been documented (Box 6.2) but the ideal may be far from the reality. The need to develop and promote a supportive working context is an ongoing process before, during and following engagement in an action research study.

Box 6.2

Contextual requirements for collaboration (Henneman et al. 1995)

- Visionary leaders supportive of autonomy
- Recognition of the boundaries of one's discipline
- A team orientation with effective group dynamics
- Organisational values which include participation and interdependence

Collaboration challenges

Key challenges in establishing collaboration were previously identified by Huxham (1996) (see Box 6.3).

Box 6.3

Key challenges in establishing collaboration (Huxham 1996)

1. Differences in aims, language, procedures, culture and perceived power
2. The tension between autonomy and accountability and the lack of authority
3. The time needed to manage the logistics:
   - actual time invested in achieving mutual understanding, gaining goodwill, negotiating bases for action and coordination (all of which are related to creating trust)
   - lapsed time to cope with accountability issues and organisational priorities

The need to find common ground with all healthcare colleagues, managers and patients requires a process of dialogue and cooperation (Koch and Kralik 2006). Yet, the difficulty of establishing collaboration in an Intensive Care Unit, where it is often assumed there are close working relationships, is revealed by La Pine (2008). In her action research project, she bemoans the fact that the advantages of collaboration are not adequately emphasised in medical education or medical practice. Difficulties of medical collaboration need to be borne in mind when considering potential barriers to change, but sometimes they may be imagined rather than be real issues. For example, the co-researchers on a surgical ward believed that medical support would not be forthcoming for their identified innovation – to systematically plan, implement and evaluate patient self-medication. Box 6.4 demonstrates the assumptions of the Ward Sister/co-researcher regarding the medical staff's reaction to the innovation, my responses as action researcher/facilitator, and the actual collaborative response from a physician.

Box 6.4

Unanticipated medical collaboration for patient self-medication proposal (Bellman 2003: 108)

Day sister (co-researcher):	'Quite honestly I don't think it's worth giving a copy [of the patient self-medication proposal] to the consultants as they'll just put it in the bin.'

Loretta (action researcher/facilitator):	'Although Mr Y [consultant surgeon] will eventually get one as he's the chair of the Drug Committee.'
Day sister:	'Oh yes but he'll pull it apart.'
Loretta:	'But it might be useful for him to pull it apart as we have a couple of weeks to play with before the next committee meets.'

A general discussion ensued. I (as action researcher/facilitator) was faced with a dilemma. I felt that although the consultants had agreed in principle, we all knew, although it was never voiced, that such is their power that any one of them could have stalled or even halted the process. The co-researchers, although having agreed and written the proposal, were still aware of this potentially restraining force. Sister agreed to distribute the proposal and at the following co-researcher meeting she produced a very supportive letter from Mr Y:

Dear Sister,

Proposal for self-medication

This looks absolutely great and I am 100% behind you. I would actually like to introduce it universally throughout the Unit, rather than wait for the pilot studies, but it may be that we will have to persuade a few people before the introduction.

If there is any way in which I can help, other than through the Drug & Therapeutics Committee, please let me know.

You are quite right that as medical and nursing staff we owe our patients a duty of care and a pre-requisite of allowing self-medication is a formal assessment and record showing that the patient is competent and capable of managing the procedure.

In the ward environment, it is certainly possible that other patients or visitors can have access to such drugs, and if loss or damage occurs as a result, the Authority would be legally liable. In order to minimise this risk, patients who are allowed to administer their own drugs must be provided with a locked drawer or cupboard in which the medicines can be kept and the patient made responsible for the custody and safe-keeping of the key.

Yours sincerely

xxxx

Chairman

Drug & Therapeutics Committee

Key messages for collaborative practice include always challenging and checking assumptions, and recognising that collaboration between all healthcare professionals takes time and that new skills may have to be learned (Coeling and Wilcox 1994). The importance of initiating and sustaining collaboration and the resultant learning should be clearly documented in action research studies. According to Hockley (2006), it is important to identify the scope of collaboration between the action researcher and the co-researchers, as collaboration can range from informing a review and diagnosis of a particular problem to identification of solutions, and the testing and evaluation of that solution in practice.

• • • REFLECTIVE EXERCISE 6.2 • • •

What challenges can you identify in establishing collaboration with colleagues, patients, carers and other key stakeholders? What needs to change in your clinical area to effectively engage in collaborative practice?

Achieving consensus

Although consensus is sometimes difficult to attain, it is a powerful instrument for change when it is achieved (Stringer 2007). Consequently, a key leadership skill for the action researcher is the ability to build a consensus, a shared vision and commitment to action, even where there may be initial disagreement. Three levels of disagreement have been categorised by Wilkinson (2010; see Box 6.5).

Box 6.5

Identifying the difficulties in reaching a consensus (Wilkinson 2010)

Why do people disagree?

People tend to disagree for one of three reasons generally, and more often than not, due to the first reason below:

1. They have not clearly heard and understood the other's alternative and reasons for supporting the alternative **(Level 1: They are not hearing each other)**
2. They have heard and understood, but they have had different experiences or hold different values that result in preferring one alternative to the other **(Level 2: They have different values or experiences)**
3. The disagreement is based on personality, past history with one another or other factors (e.g. politico-economic) that have nothing to do with the alternatives **(Level 3: Outside factors)**

Leadership skills of relationship-building also underpin the consensus process, particularly being willing to create dialogue and recognising that values will describe the parameters for initiatives and strategy (Malby 1997). In my role as lecturer/action research facilitator I shared my personal beliefs with the co-researchers:

- learning and knowledge development are most meaningful when they occur in clinical practice;
- practitioners have a wealth of practice knowledge which is of equal value to theoretical knowledge;
- the sharing of knowledge will help to enhance patient care, reduce the theory–practice gap and develop nursing knowledge;
- in recognition of, and to develop, practitioners' clinical expertise and professional judgement they should be enabled and feel empowered to make changes for patient benefit (Bellman 1996: 132).

Hockley (2006; see also Nolan and Grant 1993) recognised that the action researcher pays particular attention to helping collaborators question and critically reflect on the 'values' that underpin their practice when bringing about change. In the exploratory phase of her study to develop and improve the quality of end-of-life care for residents in two independent nursing homes, staff talked about what they found difficult and how they thought end-of-life care might be developed. There was little explicit challenge to the staff values that underpinned the care of a dying resident. However, the drawing out of basic values about the area undergoing change, and the clarifying of values across staff groups, became important as the study progressed. A match between what we say we believe and what we do is one of the hallmarks of effective individuals, teams and organisations (Manley 2000). By facilitating regular group sessions, Hockley (2006) noted that staff showed an increasing willingness to share their own values about end-of-life care and then together identified how they wanted them implemented in practice.

Participants' values may emerge over time, as for Hockley (2006). Other action research studies have involved the sharing of values at the commencement of a project. For example, in the Recovery area of the operating theatres, I and two co-facilitators (Bellman et al. 2003) commenced the project by undertaking a values clarification exercise (see Box 6.6) to explore the basis of our collaboration (i.e. our values regarding practice development) for individual nurses, the clinical team, the organisation, and the extent of user involvement.

Box 6.6

Values clarification exercise (Manley 1992)

A values clarification exercise is a grand title for a simple exercise designed to access and clarify the values and beliefs we hold about something. It always starts with a stem to help identify the main/ultimate purpose. For example, 'I/we believe the ultimate purpose of x is……'. This stem would always be followed by a second stem which identifies how the purpose can be achieved. For example, 'I/we believe this purpose can be achieved by….'. A number of other stems would usually be included depending on the purpose of the exercise. Key to developing and realising a common shared vision is the involvement of as many stakeholders as possible in the process.

For the purpose of developing a shared understanding of practice development, for example, the following stems may be useful:

- I believe the ultimate purpose of practice development is ……..
- I believe this purpose can be achieved by ……..
- I believe my role is ……..
- I believe the factors that inhibit or enable this purpose to be achieved include: ……..
- Other values/beliefs that I hold about practice development are ……..

We then used the values clarification exercise to explore and reflect with the co-researchers the ultimate purpose of Recovery Room Nursing. We also explored the nature of support for one another and the co-researchers, and identified the need for ongoing support for the project, particularly from senior managers.

Street (2008) conducted an action research inquiry into the transfer of knowledge from a continuing education course on pain interventions into clinical practice. She found that it was the experienced, knowledgeable and confident healthcare professionals/co-researchers who were more able to build a consensus for change. Reflecting on her project, she identified three main 'conditions' for collaboration (see Box 6.7).

Box 6.7

Reflecting on the three main conditions for collaboration (Street 2008: 292–293)

1 The first condition was to enable and identify an improved knowledge base (of pain management) and the confidence to access evidence based sources.
2 I found that the collective impact on practice was greatest when nurses from this study were able to work together and support each other with practice initiatives. Characteristically, there will always be external pressures and

changes within health care. Even within the timeframe of this research, external events occurred which made a significant impact on the (pain) interventions some of the nurses elected to pursue. Because action research is concerned with an understanding of the conditions in which practice occurs, the flexibility of this approach to inquiry is, I suggest, relevant to the health care context. This conviction is shared by Waterman et al. (2001: 52), who commend action researchers' ability to be responsive and flexible and provide feedback in complex social situations. Reflecting this flexibility, the nurses were able to act on unexpected opportunities to improve aspects of (pain) care.

3. I found that the nurses' perceived level of practice influence was inextricably linked to their experience. Nurses who were more recently qualified found it more difficult to challenge decisions that they were unhappy about and described circumstances where more experienced colleagues disregarded their opinions. A few nurses also experienced anti-intellectual comments from their practice colleagues. It appears, therefore, that even when nurses have the knowledge they may not always have the authority to change practice.
4. The overall outcome of enhanced collaboration and improved communication was a reduction in nurses' perception of practice barriers to pain care. By changing their own practice, and becoming less critical of others, they lessened the effect of some practice barriers they had previously attributed to colleagues' behaviours rather than their own.

• • • REFLECTIVE EXERCISE 6.3 • • •

Consider the content of Boxes 6.6 and 6.7. How may this information support your project in your own clinical setting?

Facilitation

Effective facilitation, when working with individuals and teams, is an essential component of carrying out action research. Facilitation does not happen by 'accident'. Instead it is an intentional, skilled act that needs to underpin both individual and group learning. Within the past decade the literature on facilitation has increased substantially to enable a better understanding of the concept in a variety of contexts (education, research, health, practice development and counselling), leading to a number of interpretations, desired attributes and outcomes (Harvey et al. 2002; Lambert and Glacken 2005; Manley et al. 2008). In addition a number of models, frameworks and standards have been developed to enable a better understanding of facilitation (Heron 1989; Hersey and Blanchard 1996; Royal College of Nursing 2005) aimed at supporting those involved with facilitation at both a micro and macro level. Also, facilitation aimed at enabling reflection through critical companionship (Titchen 2000) and active learning (Dewing 2008, 2009) have focused upon learning in and from practice in which the facilitator is an 'active learner' along with those being facilitated. Within the action research literature this is key, as the facilitator will enable action as a consequence of learning within the action research cycle. Heron (1989) identifies six dimensions of facilitation and three styles of intervention (see Box 6.8). Heron suggests that the facilitator should be able to work within any of the dimensions, applying different styles of intervention depending on the context and need at that time.

Box 6.8

Facilitation dimensions and intervention (Heron 1989)

Six dimensions of facilitation

- **Planning** – how the group manages itself and allocated resources
- **Meaning** – how the group understands group processes and learning from the context
- **Confronting** – feelings, assumptions, objective and subjective interpretations
- **Feeling** – being able to work with feelings; conscious control of emotional processes and methods
- **Structuring** – the session, presentation and how participants are able to engage in learning (group and individual)
- **Valuing** – others, self, learning, patients and group processes

Three styles of intervention

- **Hierarchy** – the facilitator is responsible for all decision making and subsequent action
- **Cooperation** – working collaboratively between the facilitator and individuals in decision making
- **Autonomy** – decision making and responsibility for decision making is devolved to the individual

••• REFLECTIVE EXERCISE 6.4 •••

Consider your current role as a facilitator. Can you identify with the six dimensions of facilitation and three styles of intervention in Box 6.8?

The skills and attributes needed to help individuals develop within their role as an effective facilitator, with individuals, teams and within the broader organisational context, remains at times varied and not always valued as a whole. For example, Burrows (1997: 403) suggests that if educators are to view facilitation as more than a mere resource, they must develop their practice and evaluate their skills in order to implement facilitation competently and confidently. Indeed, all potential facilitators need to appreciate that facilitation is a complex process which requires skill, insight and support. Insight into the complexity of the role is provided in Box 6.9.

Box 6.9

Reflections of an action researcher facilitator (Weaver and Nicholls 2001: 182)

As a facilitator I often felt very nervous. I was nervous of the responsibility and I struggled with the idea of being the facilitator and therefore having a degree of power. I thought, God, this is all being tape-recorded, and is part of a research project which may be circulated to lots of mental health organisations. It felt like really big stuff for me, very grand. But at the same time I really wanted to do it, and thought, well, you know, perhaps it's going to be all right. And on the whole it was.

The power issue is very complicated. For example, we may not necessarily feel powerful in relation to the group of people we are working with, but to them we may *appear* powerful. Even though we may feel anxious and unskilful, to the other people in the group we're coming in with a 'researcher' hat on and that may have connotations for some of them.

• • • REFLECTIVE EXERCISE 6.5 • • •

What skills, insight and support would you consider essential for developing the role of facilitator for your action research project?

While there are core skills, such as interpersonal and communication skills, that are prerequisites for any facilitator role, it appears that to be effective, facilitators require a number of skills and personal attributes, depending on the context and purpose (Rycroft-Malone et al. 2004: 174). In a concept analysis of facilitation, Burrows (1997) identifies four critical attributes for effective facilitation (see Box 6.10).

Box 6.10

A synopsis of four critical attributes for effective facilitation (Burrows 1997)

Genuine mutual respect – to achieve genuine mutual respect, facilitators must create an open learning climate in which participants are able to share their thoughts and feelings.

A partnership in learning – the partnership involves the facilitator as a co-learner. The facilitator either takes or delegates leadership, but responsibility is shared through a process of negotiation.

A dynamic goal-orientated process – facilitation is proactive and dynamic. The process involves assisting with goal identification, encouraging investigation, giving meaning to activities and indicating appropriate resources.

Practice of critical reflection – facilitators should promote strategies of questioning, probing and debating so that learners are able to question their own and others' assumptions, thoughts and attitudes.

Implementing these critical attributes in clinical action research projects can be, at times, extremely challenging, often due to time constraints within co-researcher meetings. Yet, the facilitator of an action research project is seen by Winter and Munn-Giddings (2001: 43) as a focus for the activity within the project, providing emotional support, practice assistance, and acting as a resource, critic, recorder of the project, and methodological teacher.

Within the practice development literature, which often utilises action research methodology, skilled facilitation is a key element in transforming both practitioners and practice (Manley et al. 2008; McCormack et al. 2006). Hence, in considering the place of facilitation within the context of 'enabling' clinical change and practice development, Shaw et al. (2008) identify six key factors that emerged as consequences or outcomes for the concept of enabling (see Box 6.11).

Box 6.11

A synopsis of the consequences or outcomes for the concept of enabling (Shaw et al. 2008)

Interdependence – in practice development it is important to achieve a balance between independence and being influenced by others. Interdependence relates to working collaboratively with others within agreed values and beliefs to achieve a shared vision.

Collaborative leading – to enable teams to work effectively, a facilitator must first establish what the culture they are working in is and gain a consensus of what the cultural norms are.

Responsibility for learning, growth and development – through learning for oneself, it is important that learning is used, and seen to be used, by other stakeholders and out into action.

Value, validation and self-worth – central to being enabled is the importance of feeling valued, validation and self-worth.

Vision and perspective – having a common, agreed vision across stakeholders is key to ensuring that there is an agreed focus and targeted outcomes.

Action oriented – creating possibilities is necessary as part of vision creation and seeing perspectives. This on occasions can be challenging for practitioners due to the 'trials' and 'tribulations' of day-to-day practice.

These factors can be viewed as being core to defining the enabling qualities that underpin facilitation within the context of 'transformational' and/or emancipatory intent. Achieving emancipatory intent is a fundamental principle within many action research studies. According to Piggot-Irvine and Bartlett (2005), the more participative the project leadership, the more emancipatory its effects may become. This is because the facilitator proceeds on the basis of developing involvement and shared commitment rather than disempowering participants through, for example, hierarchical control or unilateral decision making. To avoid participants feeling manipulated (Searson 2001), to ensure that multiple perspectives are elicited, and that forceful people do not dominate proceedings, the facilitator should employ judicious, diplomatic, yet firm processes, providing participants with opportunities to articulate their thoughts and ideas in safety (Stringer 2007).

Winter and Munn-Giddings (2001: 43) also caution that while an action research project is always attempting to overcome authority and dependency, a well-intentioned facilitator may produce unintended dependency and a hierarchical power relationship. For example, three project co-facilitators, a Nurse Unit Manager, Research Assistant and Professor of Nursing Research and Practice Development, assumed that what they perceived as a problem, underpinned by a wealth of research evidence, would automatically be perceived as a problem to be collaboratively resolved by their clinical colleagues (Smith et al. 2009). This assumption had a disempowering effect on potential participants and initially inhibited stakeholder consultation.

In exploring the role of the facilitator and the context of facilitation, Harvey et al. (2002) describe a hands-on approach to facilitating change in complex, multidimensional settings, in which there is a greater focus on helping rather than persuading or instructing (Aggergaard Larsen et al. 2005: 147). As a Ward Sister, Kennedy (2001) used this approach to empower a second-year student (who identified the innovation) and her ward team to undertake initial literature searches and follow-up discussions at ward meetings followed by collaborative change. The concept of *participative facilitation* encompasses a hands-on approach and was identified as part of an integrative framework for clinical change and development (Chapter 3) (Bellman 2003). Box 6.12 reflects the participative facilitation process (see also Chapter 4).

Box 6.12

Participative facilitation (Bellman 2003)

- Be familiar with the action research, change and practice development literature.
- Enlist managers' ongoing support and participation.
- Negotiate an appropriate environment for group meetings.
- Explore the organisational culture in regard to:
  - practice development
  - innovative change
  - patient/user involvement
  - intra-professional and multi-professional collaboration.
- Ensure co-researchers' initial and ongoing consent to participate.
- Define the roles of the action researcher/facilitator and co-researchers.
- Value each co-researcher's contribution.
- Encourage exploration of patient-focused problems/issues.
- Establish group consensus/negotiated agreement for identified change.
- Enlist multi-professional cooperation and collaboration.
- Establish ongoing action plans within realistic timeframes.
- Ensure the identification of empowering processes and support for disempowering processes.
- Undertake process and outcome evaluations.
- Participate in collaborative report writing.

Key questions for the facilitator to consider are:

1. How does the action research facilitator provide support without taking control?
2. How does the facilitator provide a critical perspective and encourage participants to have confidence in their own experience?
3. How can the 'pressure' provided by the facilitator's presence be 'stimulating' rather than 'inhibiting'? (Messner and Rauch 1995)
4. How does the facilitator enable rather than 'direct' anticipated outcomes?

• • • REFLECTIVE EXERCISE 6.6 • • •

Consider how you would you tackle points 1–4 above in your action research project. Some perspectives within a narrative account are provided in the journey of facilitation below.

Facilitation in practice

The facilitation literature provides the action researcher with insight into the complexity, challenges and rewards of the facilitation process. Narrative accounts are equally informative. The following narrative describes an action research project in which the facilitator/Consultant Nurse for Older People worked with a group of five Registered Nurses (the participants) as part of an emancipatory practice development programme. The aim of the programme was to develop person-centred assessment with older people. The programme ran for two and a half years in a District General Hospital (Webster 2007, 2009). The narrative will describe action research Cycle Two, of Phase 3 of the study, in which the facilitator met with the participants for two hours once every two weeks over a four-month period to explore the meaning and implementation of 'assessment' when undertaken with older people.

The journey of facilitation

Five Registered Nurses from acute and specialist general medical wards had been nominated to take part in the programme: one from ward C1, three from ward C3 and one from ward C4. I was uncertain why only one person alone had been nominated from C4. When I spoke with the Senior Nurse for C4 I was told that due to other commitments, it was only possible to release one member of staff from this clinical area to take part in the project at that time. I sensed that C4 was no longer committed to the programme as, although it was not openly stated, the focus of the programme was perceived as being of no value or relevance to this clinical area, although initially support had been forthcoming. Also, I was acutely aware of the limitations of my role as a facilitator as I was working as an 'outsider' to the team and that ownership needed to come from within the senior team on C4. I recognised that I could only support C4 if they were willing to work with me. Subsequently, the participant from C4 stopped attending after three sessions. I made various attempts to make contact but received no response.

Early on I became aware that the participants were unsure of what to expect both in the sessions and in regard to their role in sharing their learning with colleagues. This highlighted a lack of clarity on my part in my initial preparations. It soon became clear that the participants viewed the programme as focusing solely on their own individual development. In fact, the objectives of the programme were threefold, to focus on:

- their professional development;
- the development of colleagues;
- practice development within their own clinical settings.

On reflection I should have realised that I would have acquired greater clarity and understanding of both their work-based culture and the values underpinning their own practice if I had initially seen the world 'through their eyes'. I needed to enable participants to both explore and articulate the key opportunities and clinical challenges they experienced working with older people in an acute hospital setting.

To address the lack of clarity I reaffirmed the values underpinning the programme. This reinforced that the programme was an evolutionary journey both for me as a facilitator and for the participants. We were all gaining greater insight and understanding into different areas of practice with older people. For me, as a facilitator, I was conscious that I was gaining greater insight and understanding of the complexities of clinical practice and the elements that both enable and inhibit creative, person-centred practice with older people. Underpinning this, I recognised that as a facilitator I was moving between the six dimensions of facilitation and three styles of intervention (Heron 1989; Box 6.8), depending on the context and individual needs at that time. I was also applying the six categories of intervention in how I worked with and facilitated individuals (see Box 6.13). I shared my insights with the group and agreed with the participants to undertake ongoing process evaluations with them regarding their professional development, their experience of the programme, including practice change and innovation, and their feedback regarding the facilitation process.

Box 6.13

Six categories of intervention (Heron 1989)

- **Prescriptive interventions** – the facilitator suggests or recommends particular actions or approaches. This may include recommendations related to behaviours, reflection or literature to read related to practice.
- **Informative interventions** – the facilitator informs or directs the person. Over-use of this approach can lead the person to become dependent on the facilitator.

- **Confronting interventions** – the person is challenged by the facilitator or draws their attention to a particular behaviour (this needs to be balanced against supportive interventions).
- **Cathartic interventions** – the facilitator enables the person to release 'tension' through expression of their feelings. NB: the facilitator needs to be able to facilitate such emotions and the translation into positive action.
- **Catalytic interventions** – the facilitator draws the person out, enabling them to develop understanding and encouraging them to discuss issues further.
- **Supportive interventions** – the facilitator supports, validates and encourages the person.

'Person' refers to practitioner, clinician or participant.

Another uncertainty I had regarding the facilitation process was how I was perceived by the participants. We had agreed to undertake reflective exercises between meetings. However, frequently the co-researchers would refer to the reflective exercises as being homework. I questioned this use of terminology as I did not perceive it as being work that I would check as being right or wrong. I also felt a degree of anxiety as I was uncertain as to whether those taking part perceived me as a traditional teacher rather than a contemporary enabler who was enabling them to critically reflect upon their own practice while developing greater knowledge and understanding of the process of person-centred assessment with older people. The literature had enabled me to appreciate the strengths and differences between technical and emancipatory approaches. For example, Manley and McCormack (2004) identify that a technical approach is focused on gaining technical knowledge that will enable greater mastery and skill over technical work whereas an emancipatory approach is focused on transforming the culture and context of care in which practitioners feel empowered to not only critically question and challenge, but to change and develop practice. I therefore tried to enable the group by using different approaches in sensitive, supportive and challenging ways. I facilitated in equal measure direct questioning and challenging of each other as well as being openly supportive and reflective. This did not necessarily provide all the answers or solutions, but I was encouraged to see the group, with my support, emulating these approaches.

It was inevitable that organisational needs would sometimes impact on this phase of the programme. As a facilitator, I needed to establish clear structural parameters. For this reason we agreed that if only two people could attend the session it would be rescheduled. The timing of the sessions was also changed to better accommodate the clinical requirements of the areas taking part, i.e. those areas taking part were under extreme pressure as a result of clinical activity and therefore needed appropriate staffing to ensure patient safety.

As a result of the reflective exercises that the co-researchers had worked through between sessions, I was conscious at times that our meetings appeared to partly turn into what could be termed group clinical supervision sessions. On occasions we moved away from the main theme of focus for that day. However, in facilitating the group I felt that these *significant reflective digressions* were appropriate as group members were critically reflecting upon occurrences from their practice that had been triggered by the reflective exercise. I was aware that frequently I used transferable skills developed through my past experience of clinical supervision and critical companionship (Titchen 2000) to facilitate reflection. This enabled me to recognise that follow-up support was also needed for some individuals, i.e. talking through specific, sensitive issues or concerns that may have emerged in the session. Increasingly within the group, the members sought validation and support from their peers. I was conscious that my role as a facilitator changed as group members increasingly facilitated one another through critical questioning and support. I was thankful that this change in the group over a period of time marked the transition from which I was perceived less as a traditional teacher and more as both co-facilitator and co-traveller on a shared journey of innovation and development.

Increasingly, the examples that participants brought from practice were more in-depth and complex (compared with their initial more superficial reflections). Group members also appeared to be more critically reflective of their practice and were becoming more systematic in their documentation and descriptions of the critically reflective approach that they took. Reflection-in-action (Schön 1999) became more common place. Heidi stated at one session:

> I was caring for an older man who had been admitted on my shift. I thought about what we had talked about and how important it was to find out about people. I sensed that something wasn't right. He was acutely ill, but there was something else. I asked him what was important to him and he identified that he was worried about who would feed his dog while he was in hospital ... it was something really small and not what I had expected. However we sorted it out and he appeared more relaxed. It helped me to see him, what was important to him, rather than an old man who was ill!

Reflection-in-action can be seen as involving two distinct components. First, the ability to turn thought back on action so that the practitioner is aware of *what* they are doing. Second, to consider *how* they are doing it, demonstrating practical knowledge that is underpinning practice (Rolfe et al. 2001: 19). Heidi demonstrated this level of understanding based on her account. She knew that 'something wasn't right' and used the knowledge she had gained from the session to make sense of her observations and the subsequent development of an informed plan of action. I found illustrations such as this very exciting and they invigorated the sessions. A synthesis of creative thinking resulted from group discussion and facilitation which enabled participants to start working in a greater person-centred way with older people. However, I was conscious that illustrations such as Heidi's might be perceived as being light-weight by the other participants. Yet, they were the key to illustrating a greater person-centred approach to assessment with older people.

I observed that as the sessions progressed a strong sense of support and cohesion was developing among the group. I became increasingly aware that the co-researchers were very committed to taking part and would attend even if they had been rostered as a day off. This level of commitment and subsequent energy from the group was evident throughout this whole phase and was reflected in the ownership of the programme as we progressed.

Likewise I felt that I was being viewed differently by those taking part. The initial view of him and us had changed to a far greater sense of mutuality based on joint learning and development. On occasions, discussions became highly energised, and as a participative facilitator it was exciting to be part of them. Also I could see how individuals had grown, including ways in which group members were now supporting one other. At the end of this phase I observed that participants had travelled a long way in developing a greater understanding of the process of person-centred assessment with older people. I naturally felt a degree of responsibility for this change, but also an increasing unease. Frequently, within the group discussion we had focused on ways of influencing colleagues and the challenges associated with changing practice, especially when others may be resistant or cynical of the change. At this stage I was unsure how supportive the organisational culture would be to the participants and whether current systems would enable them to influence colleagues and subsequently develop practice. However, as a result of the programme, other collaborative work grew and evolved with participants and participating areas, such as taking forward the outcomes of observations of care and using patient stories to develop practice with older people.

Learning from the journey of facilitation

There was much learning that came from this example of working with the group. Rycroft-Malone et al. (2002: 82) identify that effective facilitation needs to match the purpose, role and skills needed by a certain situation. While working with the group I found myself adapting how I worked with them, depending on the context and the needs of both participants and the group at that time. I was clear about the purpose of the meetings. However, at times I needed to be flexible, depending on the variety of different needs and organisational requirements impacting on participants. Facilitation in the real-world context is challenging and as a facilitator I found that I was constantly drawing from both empirical and experiential knowledge as I creatively worked with different situations and challenges. In doing so, I moved between the three styles of intervention: hierarchy, cooperation and autonomy (Heron 1989). Similarly, the work-based setting can be less than ideal due to the many pressures that participants faced on a day-to-day basis. For this reason, as a facilitator, I needed to show great flexibility, along with the ability to adapt and seize opportunities, as I knew that if I waited for the ideal, this may never occur.

• • • REFLECTIVE EXERCISE 6.7 • • •

Consider an occasion when you facilitated a group or individual. What worked well? What would you do differently in the future?

Clinical academic collaboration and facilitation

Learning to use research in clinical practice is now an international clinical objective within postgraduate nurse education (Forsman et al. 2009). The literature recognises the collaborative role of educators and researchers as:

- leading and supporting a research-based culture for practice (Girot 2010);
- being important facilitators of research use in the healthcare system (Profetto-McGrath et al. 2008: 207);
- supporting nurses and improving the research environment (Pringle 1989);
- seeing a research project not as a goal in itself but as a method to achieve broader goals:
  - learning knowledge and skills relevant to the task in hand,
  - developing relationships of solidarity, and
  - engaging in action that wins victories and builds self-sufficiency (Stoecker 2008: 845).

The development of a collaborative research relationship between a hospital Trust and university is relatively new (Jinks and Green 2004). In an action research study to introduce bedside handovers, Searson (2001: 86), a university lecturer, concluded that the nurses in the Coronary Care Unit wanted help with the research process – something they didn't think was available at that time. There are now increasing opportunities for clinical academic collaboration and facilitation. For example, a more recent study provides greater insight into the collaboration and facilitation process between two university lecturers and a research and practice development nurse (Crow et al. 2006).

The three authors use the analogy of journeying into unfamiliar territory to convey their experience of moving between cultures to establish collaboration across the academic and healthcare organisations. The focus of their action research project was to raise awareness of and improve practice for all staff regarding dignity and respect shown to patients and their visitors in hospital. The authors considered that the mode of action research they employed moved from an initial practical/technical approach to a more critical/emancipatory approach. The critical conversations that they had had shaped the development of the project and could be seen to achieve a communicative space (see Chapter 4). They documented in their reflective diaries the challenges that occurred within their collaborative approach. For example, a snapshot from the first phase of the project, which involved the development and evaluation of a new dignity and respect university programme, revealed the following challenges:

- While the lecturers were on familiar ground, the nurse had to adjust from a clinical environment, where quick solutions to practical problems were routine, to what was seen as a slower pace of work with a focus on discussion, debate and reflection.
- To reach a utilitarian consensus for the greater good, the lecturers had to compromise their philosophy of democratic education and acknowledge the nurse's perspective regarding the hospital's culture and resultant expectation for the programme.
- The nurse reluctantly acquiesced to the lecturers' proposal for dealing with a participant's inappropriate conduct in the classroom. The nurse would have proceeded along a formal disciplinary route. The issue made the educators reflect on precisely whose interest they were protecting – students or service users/patients.
- In Phase 2, implementing change in practice, the lecturers discussed feelings of unease, low autonomy and fear that their journey was now being controlled by other, more powerful agents and agendas in the hospital. The nurse was more adept at 'cutting paths through the forests of bureaucracy' (Crow et al. 2006: 302).

Overall, as insider/outsider action researchers, all three recognised the extent to which they had supported each other while working in what they perceived to be alien territory, and acknowledged the shared learning as well as the complementary knowledge and skills that each had brought to the project.

Collaboration and facilitation across organisations enables new, more appropriate ways of working, including challenging the status quo, norms and assumptions. For the lecturers, this also included a recognised norm in that many educators of health professionals teach their students in the university and then send them back into the clinical setting to implement changes. There may be many reasons for this, including excessive teaching workload, lack of confidence in clinical settings, research knowledge gaps, and disinterest in research/knowledge application in practice.

According to Jinks and Green (2004), there are university infrastructures which are designed to help and enhance the research skills of staff members. These authors also report that in their university, opportunities exist to reduce a teaching workload while undertaking a research secondment. However, they report that there was limited interest by lecturers to undertake a research project. Yet, for the lecturers in the Crow et al. (2006) project, the experience of co-facilitating an action research project for patient benefit directly influenced their teaching. There was also an increased understanding of the ubiquitous gap between classroom theories and transforming practice, and of the so-called 'rush rush' environment of the hospital where there is often limited space for staff to transform their understanding of self or explore how their work situation influences their assumptions and behaviours.

The focus on the benefits of collaboration could lead one to think that collaboration is a favorite approach to providing patient care, leading organisations, educating future health professionals, and conducting healthcare research (Gardner 2005). While the benefits are clearly evident, there are many challenging elements, including establishing effective dialogue, consensus-building and overcoming clinical academic boundaries. Both strategic and operational clinical academic challenges were evident in a hospital-wide action research project (Bellman and Wiseman 2010). Perspectives of both clinical and academic staff led to the identification of a key theme: academic input into practice-based research (see Box 6.14). The theme demonstrates the need for clinical academic co-leadership, facilitation and shared learning for the realistic development and advancement of practice-based research. Also clearly evident is the need for greater cohesion and integration of university research programmes to support practice-based research.

Box 6.14

Examples from the theme: academic input into practice-based research (Bellman and Wiseman 2010)

Research is seen as university-driven and remote from the care setting:

> The degree course gives you all the information but then you don't necessarily know how to take the most relevant bits to use in practice. (Clinical Nurse Specialist)
>
> You spend all that time doing a fantastic literature review but then that's it. ... I think some of it does come down to the way that the lecturers are divorced from the practicalities on the ward. (Divisional Senior Nurse)
>
> Looking at the pre-reg. curriculum ... research and the application of its findings and evaluation of research is low profile within the curriculum. So already there is, I think, a mindset. (Senior Clinical Nurse)
>
> In this clinical area we're looking at the evidence that underpins our practice. We need some support in how do we acquire advanced literature skills etc., and then how to look at and analyze the literature, and then how to get the evidence into practice. I could see us working together with a lecturer. (Clinical Nurse Specialist)
>
> If you've been an academic for a while, you're a support, a resource, you could run a journal club, encourage people to look at different evidence. Let's explore ways of putting this into practice, support somebody doing their Masters degree on this particular ward ... they need to be visible with our support. (Divisional Senior Nurse)
>
> It's taking those key people [in the university] who are currently doing a participatory type of research out in the clinical practice areas and really promoting that. Showing researchers in the university that are coming up, but also those in the clinical departments who want to do research, that that's a way that they can all work together. (Academic Executive)
>
> The focus in university really has to change to the patient pathway and meeting the needs of patients. There's the need to extend that pathway into the community as we need to equip nurses with the ability to move between areas. (Divisional Senior Nurse)
>
> There will be skills that the clinical staff have got around research that the academic staff don't have. So I don't think it should always be seen as all of the knowledge and skills lie with the university because I think there's far more based in the Trusts and the Community than some of the [academic] staff realise they've got. (Academic Executive)
>
> There's no reason why we couldn't have joint clinical academic appointments in nursing with our local universities, as we do with medical appointments. (Executive Manager)

(Continued)

> *(Continued)*
>
> So it is a culture of getting some people [in the university] to realise that research doesn't have to be 'I've got a grant from the Medical Research Council etc. for funding for the next three years for research fellows'. Some of it is about what is your day-to-day work. You need to research what's out there, what's written in the current journals, what's the current practice out in the Trust. That can then also be brought back into the university for teaching the students and to develop the new curriculum. (Academic Executive)

Summary

A key part of the knowledge base for conducting an action research project in clinical practice is an understanding of collaboration. Also essential is an understanding of the strengths and challenges of the facilitation process, together with developing the skills needed to facilitate. Too often the skills needed to facilitate groups and individuals effectively can go unrecognised or are not valued. Participative facilitation enables shared learning and reflective experiences to develop and advance professional knowledge and practice, for both participants and facilitator. Building a consensus and a shared commitment to action can be a challenging process. Flexible working and ongoing organisational support are required and a key component is commitment to the process of enabling both practitioners and practice to develop. Academic input into practice-based research is an essential collaborative process to support the application of research knowledge in practice, the sharing of theoretical and experiential knowledge, the development of contemporary research curricula and so much more. In addition, the skills and wealth of experience of practitioners who work with and care for people in the real-world context should not be undervalued as ultimately they will translate knowledge and make improved outcomes a reality for patients.

Useful websites

Foundation of Nursing Studies (FoNS), Centre for nursing innovation: www.fons.org/ offers support in undertaking the collaboration and facilitation process.

Resources for facilitators: www.managementhelp.org/grp_skll/resource.htm provides a wealth of online information.

References

Aggergaard Larsen, J, Maundrill, R, Morgan, J and Moulans, L (2005) Practice development facilitation: An integrated strategic and clinical approach. *Practice Development in Health Care* 4(3): 142–149.

Argyris, C, Putnam, R and Smith, D (1985) *Action science*. San Francisco, CA: Jossey-Bass.

Bellman, L (1996) Changing nursing practice through reflection on the Roper, Logan and Tierney model: The enhancement approach to action research. *Journal of Advanced Nursing* 24: 129–138.

Bellman, L (2003) *Nurse-led change and development in clinical practice*. Nursing Research Series. London: Wiley-Blackwell.

Bellman L & Wiseman T. (2010) Exploring Nurse/Midwifery Leadership in Using & Doing Research in Clinical Practice: Phase 1. University College London Hospitals NHS Foundation Trust, unpublished report.

Bellman, L, Bywood, C and Dale, S (2003) Advancing working and learning through critical action research: Creativity and constraints. *Nurse Education in Practice* 3(4): 186–194.

Bellman, L and Corrigan, P (2010) Using action research to develop a thoracic support nurse role to enhance quality of care. *Nursing Times* 106 (22) (8–14 June): 18–21.

Burrows, D E (1997) Facilitation: A concept analysis. *Journal of Advanced Nursing* 25: 396–404. Article first published online on 28 June 2008. DOI: 10.1046/j.1365–2648.1997.1997025396.x.

Coeling, H V and Wilcox, J R (1994) Steps to collaboration. *Nursing Administration Quarterly* 18(4): 44–55.

Crow, J, Smith, L and Keenan, I (2006) Journeying between the education and hospital zones in a collaborative action research project. Educational Action Research14(2): 287–306.

Dewing J. (2008) Becoming and being active learners and creating active learning workplaces: the value of active learning. In McCormack B, Manley K & Wilson V (eds) *International Practice Development in Nursing and Healthcare* Blackwell Publishing, Oxford, pp. 273–294.

Dewing J (2009) Moments of movement: active learning and practice development. *Nurse Education in Practice* 10, 22–26.

Forsman, H, Gustavsson, P, Ehrenberg, A, Rudman, A and Wallin, L (2009) Research use in clinical practice: Extent and patterns among nurses one and three years post-graduation. *Journal of Advanced Nursing* 65, (6): 1195-1206) DOI: 10.1111/j.365-2648.2008.04942.x.

Gardner, D B (2005) Ten lessons in collaboration. *Online Journal of Issues in Nursing* 10(1), Manuscript 1,http://www.nursingworld.org/ojin/topic26/tpc26_1.htm (accessed 1/4/2010).

Girot, E A (2010) The challenges facing lecturers and professors to lead and promote a research-based culture for practice. *Journal of Research in Nursing* 15(3): 245–257.

Glasby, J and Dickinson, H (2008) Greater than the sum of our parts? Emerging lessons for health and social care. *International Journal of Integrated Care* 8: 1–5.

Hall, J (2006) Professionalizing action research: A meaningful strategy for modernizing services? *Journal of Nursing Management* 14: 196–200.

Henneman, E A, Lee, J L and Cohen, J I (1995) Collaboration: A concept analysis. *Journal of Advanced Nursing* 21: 103–109.

Heron, J (1989) *The facilitator's handbook*. London: Kogan Page.

Hersey, P and Blanchard, K (1996) Great ideas revisited: Revisiting the life-cycle theory of leadership. *Training and Development* 50(1): 42–76.

Hockley, J (2006) Developing high quality end-of-life care in nursing homes: An action research study. PhD thesis, University of Edinburgh and Steinberg Collection, RCN.

Huxham, C (ed.) (1996) *Creating collaborative advantage*. London: Sage.

Jinks, A M and Green, H E (2004) Clinical and academic perspectives on how to develop and enhance nursing research activities. *Nursing Times Research* 9: 401–410. DOI: 10.1177/136140960400900605.

Kennedy, N (2001) Developing nursing practice: Introducing knee-length anti-embolic stockings. In R Winter and C Munn-Giddings (eds), *A handbook for action research in health andsocial care*. London: Routledge.

Koch, T and Kralik, D (2006) *Participatory action research in healthcare*. Oxford: Blackwell.

La Pine, M P (2008) The domain of nursing: Developing practice through action research in the intensive care unit. Unpublished Master of Nursing dissertation, Victoria University of Wellington, New Zealand.

Lambert, V and Glacken, M (2005) Clinical education facilitators: A literature review. *Journal of Clinical Nursing* 14(6): 664–673.

Lindeke, LL and Sieckert, AM (2005) Nurse–physician workplace collaboration. *Online Journal of Issues in Nursing* 10(1), www.medscape.com/voewarticle/499268.

Malby, R (1997) Developing the future leaders of nursing in the UK. *European Nurse* 2(1): 27–36.

Manley, K (1992) Quality assurance: The pathway to excellence in nursing. In G Brykczinska and M Jolley (eds), *Nursing care: The challenge to change*. London: Edward Arnold.

Manley, K (2000) Organisational culture and consultant nurse outcomes: Part 1 – Organisational culture. *Nurse Critical Care* 5(4) (July–August): 179–84.

Manley, K and McCormack, B (2004) Practice development: Purpose, methodology, facilitation andevaluation. In B McCormack, K Manley and R Garbett (eds), *Practice development in nursing*. Oxford: Blackwell.

Manley, K, Webster, J, Hayle, N, Hayes, N and Minardi, H (2008) Leadership role of the consultant nurses working with older people: A co-operative enquiry. *Journal of Nursing Management* 16: 147–158.

McCormack, B, Dewar, B et al. (2006) *A realist synthesis of evidence relating to practice development: Executive summary*. Edinburgh: NHS Quality Improvement Scotland. Available online at: www.nhshealthquaility.org (last accessed 1/9/2010).

Messner, E and Rauch, F (1995) Dilemmas of facilitating action research. *Educational Action Research* 3(1): 41–53.

Nolan, M and Grant, G (1993) Action research and quality of care: A mechanism for agreeing basic values as a precursor to change. *Journal of Advanced Nursing* 18: 305–311.

Piggot-Irvine, E and Bartlett, B J (eds) (2005) *Evaluating action research*. Auckland: New Zealand Research Council.

Pringle, DM (1989) Another twist on the double helix: Research and practice. *Canadian Journal of Nursing Research* 30(4): 165–179. (Reprinted 1999)

Profetto-McGrath, J, Smith, K B, Hugo, K, Patel, A and Dussault, B (2008) Nurse educators' critical thinking dispositions and research utilization. *Nurse Education in Practice* 9: 199–208

Rolfe, G, Freshwater, D and Jasper, M (2001) *Critical reflection for nursing and the helping professions*. New York: Palgrave.

Royal College of Nursing (2006) *Accredited RCN facilitation standards*, www.rcn.org.uk/__data/assets/pdf_file/0012/203160/RCN_Accredited_Facilitation_Standards_April_2006.pdf (last accessed 1/9/2010).

Rycroft-Malone, J, Kitson, A, Harvey, G, McCormack, B, Seers, K, Titchen, A and Escibrous, C (2002) Ingredients for change: Revisiting a conceptual framework. *Quality and Safety in Healthcare* 11: 174–180.

Rycroft-Malone, J, Seers, K, Titchen, A, Harvey, G, Kitson, A and McCormack, B (2004) What counts as evidence in evidence-based practice? *Journal of Advanced Nursing* 47(1): 81–90.

Schön, D (1999) *The reflective practitioner: How professionals think in action*. Aldershot: Avebury.

Searson, F (2001) Introducing bedside handovers: Changing practice on a coronary care unit. In R Winter and C Munn-Giddings (eds), *A handbook for action research in health and social care*. London: Routledge.

Shaw, T, Dewing, J, Young, R, Devlin, M, Boomer, C and Legius, M (2008) Enabling practice development: Delving into the concept of facilitation from a practitioner perspective. In K Manley, B McCormack and V Wilson (eds), *International practice development in nursing and healthcare*. Oxford: Blackwell.

Smith, S, Lewis, P and Wilson, V (2009) A 'wee' problem: Using action research to facilitate a change in urine collection methods. *Neonatal, Paediatric and Child Health Nursing* 12(1): 15–19.

Stoecker, R (2008) Challenging institutional barriers to community-based research. *Action Research* 6(1) (March): 49–67.

Street, A (2008) An action research inquiry exploring the transfer of pain knowledge from a continuing education course into practice. PhD thesis, University of Stirling. Available online at:http://hdl.handle.net/1893/474 and Steinberg collection, RCN.

Stringer, E T (2007) *Action research: A handbook for practitioners* (3rd edition). London: Sage.

Thomas, E J, Sexton, J B and Helmreich, R L (2003) Discrepant attitudes about teamwork among critical care nurses and physicians. *Critical Care Medicine* 31(3): 956–959.

Titchen A, 2000, Professional Craft Knowledge in Patient-Centred Nursing and the Facilitation of its Development. D.Phil. Linacre College Oxford. Ashdale Press, Tackley, Oxfordshire.

Weaver, Y and Nicholls, V (2001) The Camden 'Alternative Choices in Mental Health' project. In R Winter and C Munn-Giddings (eds), *A handbook for action research in health and social care*. London: Routledge.

Webster, J (2007) Person-centred assessment with older people: An action research study to explore registered nurses' understanding of person-centred assessment within a framework of emancipatory practice development. PhD thesis, University of Portsmouth, UK.

Webster, J (2009) Expertise in practice: Older people. In S Hardt, A Titchen, B McCormack and K Manley (eds), *Revealing nursing expertise through practitioner inquiry*. Oxford: Wiley-Blackwell.

Wilkinson, M (2010) Building consensus: The art of getting to yes, www.inifac.org/articles/arconsensus.pdf (last accessed 1/9/2010).

Winter, R and Munn-Giddings, C (eds) (2001) *A handbook for action research in health and social care*. London: Routledge.

Xyrichis, A and Ream, E (2008) Teamwork: A concept analysis. *Journal of Advanced Nursing*, 61: 232–241. DOI: 10.1111/j.1365-2648.2007.04496.x.

7

ETHICAL CONSIDERATIONS

Loretta Bellman

Do I need to apply for ethical approval? This chapter will tell you why this is an essential requirement. Also, in clinical action research, many ethical considerations go beyond those required when using more traditional research approaches.

Chapter objectives

The objectives of this chapter are to:

- consider the ethical implications of engaging in clinical action research;
- identify the challenges of ethical approval for user engagement;
- explore practical approaches for ethical approval in the NHS and universities.

For colleague and user engagement the action researcher is required to consider how to ensure both equity and shared decision making throughout the study, and identify the potential personal risks (and benefits) for the co-researchers associated with the project. Three important ethical questions associated with action research are explored in this chapter:

- If researcher and participants collaborate closely, how can confidentiality and anonymity be guaranteed?
- If an action research study is a 'journey' and 'evolves', how can informed consent be meaningful?
- As action research can have political consequences, how can the researcher avoid doing harm to the participants? (Williamson and Prosser 2002: 589)

The majority of researchers who have conducted an action research project have an interesting story to share regarding the ethical approval process. Colleagues report that often neither the research application documents nor research ethics committees demonstrate an understanding of action research methodology. In this chapter, personal experience from clinical action research and evidence from the literature are shared to address current challenges.

Professional code of ethics

All qualified healthcare professionals subscribe to a professional code of ethics. For nurses and midwives, the fundamental standards of conduct, performance and ethics encompass the need to:

- treat people as individuals and respect their dignity;
- respect people's confidentiality;
- collaborate with those in your care;
- ensure informed consent;
- act in a professional manner;
- share information with colleagues;
- work effectively as part of a team;
- manage risk;
- use the best available evidence;
- keep your skills and knowledge up to date;
- keep clear and accurate records;
- act with honesty and integrity;
- deal with problems;
- uphold the reputation of your profession (NMC 2008).

••• REFLECTIVE ACTIVITY 7.1 •••

What do you consider are the differences between the NMC code and the ethical research process throughout a clinical action research project?

The code of ethics required for caring for patients is also encompassed within the ethical research process. The emphasis within research ethics is: the prevention of harm; maintaining confidentiality; ensuring informed consent; honesty and integrity; and the right to withdraw from the research project (or treatment). Two further ethical considerations when conducting an action research study, which also reflect contemporary healthcare practice, are the location of 'power' and ownership of the research. All these considerations may present challenges to both the action researcher and to the ethics committee.

Prevention of harm

Action researchers are key change agents and have a duty to protect their co-researchers (Coghlan and Brannick 2010). However, as participants often determine the direction and scope of the research, there is a fine line to tread for the action researcher between ensuring a democratic process, prevention of harm and control of the project. Box 7.1 demonstrates this fine line for the action researcher when facilitating a politically sensitive issue.

Box 7.1

Action researcher reflexivity of an ethical dilemma (Bellman 2003: 236)

The ethical dilemma for me was whether by continuing to facilitate the study I was placing the co-researchers at increasing risk of harm. With each subsequent meeting the issue of a dedicated day for children was becoming more controversial. I was concerned for their well-being. Was the study jeopardising their working relationships, especially with the Day Surgery Unit manager? The co-researchers had the right to choose whether to continue to participate in the study. Indeed, this was the ongoing informed consent agreement. I [as an outsider] could walk away from the organisation at any time, but could I risk the co-researchers being labelled as reprobates? What I had imagined may happen in a previous study – being viewed by others as problematic and divisive – was potentially becoming a reality in this study. While most of the time I sustained an outward appearance of calm, I needed regular reassurance from the co-researchers that all was well:

Rebecca: 'No I didn't get any personal flak at all.'
Loretta: 'That's good, as you know that's my constant worry.'

When the paediatric issue became politically sensitive, my apprehension and frustration increased proportionally. I tried to engender realistic expectations:

'It's a bit like "Big Brother" isn't it? At times I think this, then at others I think no, this is collaborative research! ... Hopefully it is all going to turn out well, but we don't know, and we are all in it together...'.

Prevention of harm includes co-researchers being able to participate in the study without 'subtle exploitation' (Hart and Bond 1995) or fear of retribution. A legitimate concern is how can the clinical action researcher provide assurances that the co-researchers do not feel pressurised to participate? Collaborative working (see Chapter 6) must not mask subtle exploitation by, for example, managers or academics. The researcher's need for academic achievement may override the collaborative and democratic research process and ownership of the data, the change process and outcomes. Indeed, researchers may think of participants as objects and ignore their needs (Hart and Bond 1995).

Another legitimate concern is how to facilitate the democratic approach of action research when the action researchers and not the co-researchers have chosen the focus of the project (Harrison and Brandling 2010). The perceived expert power by the co-researchers of an advanced practice nurse or lecturer as facilitator may also destabilise the democratic process. Colleagues may feel somewhat threatened as the researcher is seen as 'holding the power' because of their knowledge base (Lofman et al. 2004: 337), and for managing the research agenda.

To protect participants from 'manipulation', Williamson and Prosser (2002) propose reaching agreement with co-researchers for the transparency of project developments through both internal and external scrutiny, for example-staff meetings, public events, website information and steering groups. Ways of preventing harm were also identified within the study by Lofman et al. (2004: 336) and include:

- acting and proceeding on the co-researchers' terms;
- giving regular feedback at co-researcher review meetings;
- maintaining equal relationships by ensuring collaborative decision making;
- having awareness of expert power and different types of power (including those originally identified by French and Raven 1959);
- acting towards a common goal;
- taking personal and professional responsibility for action;
- engaging the head nurse's support in meetings;
- ensuring patients' attendance at meetings;
- identifying the achievement of patient outcomes.

Combining an organisational role with that of insider action researcher or co-researcher can be seen as potentially stressful (Williamson and Prosser 2002) and may result in personal harm. For example:

> *Co-researcher's reflective journal:* I thought I'd feel empowered with knowledge and skills to move from a functional staff nurse to a competent thoracic support nurse but I currently feel disempowered. (Bellman and Corrigan 2010: 20)

The concept of demonstrable interpersonal support (Bellman (2003) is to be found in many studies where mutual support is sought and provided by the co-researchers to one another. Clinical supervision should also be considered, and was needed for the co-researchers who experienced 'a rollercoaster of emotions and experiences' while developing a new clinical role (Bellman and Corrigan 2010: 20).

Minimising the likelihood of harm to the action researcher should be a key consideration of a research supervisor. As identified in Chapter 4, Meyer (1993) refers to the extreme isolation and self-doubt of the action researcher. Bellman (2003) experienced the transference of stress from the co-researchers to herself. The need for personal support throughout the project is discussed in Chapter 4. Also, when considering choice of research supervisor/s, it is advisable to ensure that one supervisor (particularly if there are two) has knowledge and expertise of action research. I have known colleagues to suffer personal harm, particularly needless stress and anxiety, from inappropriate research supervision. Concerns need to be shared and advice can also be sought from, for example, published action researchers, the Action Research Network for Health Care Professionals at City University, CARN (Collaborative Action Research Network) at www. mmu.ac.uk/carn and from The Foundation for Nursing Studies (FoNS) www.fons.org.

Informed consent

The nature of informed consent in action research is often viewed as controversial. While the focus of an action research project may be known at the onset, often only a tentative overview can be provided. This is because:

> Often in action research, the full implications of collaborating on a project are not known. Although people may 'sign up' to participating in an action research study, it is very difficult to know in advance exactly what action will be undertaken, because of the inductive nature of the exercise. (Hockley 2006: 70)

As action research is a journey that evolves through participation, reflection and purposeful action (Hope 1998), informed consent is a more difficult concept than in other research approaches, where studies are likely to be conceptually more developed and planned (Williamson and Prosser 2002). Both the action researcher and co-researchers take a step into the unknown (Lofman et al. 2004: 335) and may well be 'working in the dark' (Bellman 1996: 132).

In a study to develop the lecturer-practitioner (LP) role, the LP asserts that her consent could not be 'informed' as neither she nor the action researcher facilitator could know how the study would develop (Williamson and Prosser 2002: 591). As participants cannot fully know to what they are consenting when they initially agree to participate, the action researcher needs to clearly reaffirm consent at appropriate stages of the study. Munhall (2001) suggests a process consent approach where the action researcher undertakes a regular review of what the co-researchers have agreed. Hockley (2006: 98) had a similar approach to informed consent:

> At the commencement of the study in each of the nursing homes, nurse managers/owners were asked to consent to the main aim of the study with the knowledge that how practice would develop would need to be discussed further following the exploratory phase. ... In an attempt to be as transparent as possible about the research and its intention, an information sheet was clearly pinned to the notice

> board in the staff rooms in the nursing homes. Next to this there were two envelopes – one contained a handful of empty consent forms while the second was there to collect completed consent forms.

Some action researchers have not obtained written consent. In a study to analyse the roles of mental health consultant nurses, Jinks and Chalder (2007) thought that acquiring written consent was unnecessary as the participants themselves were proactive in initiating and designing the study. For Lofman et al. (2004), written informed consent was not insisted on because participating in the research was voluntary, and thus, to them, included tacit consent. The authors also believed that it would be difficult for individuals (clinical nurses in an orthopaedic ward) not to participate once the ethical committee and head nurses had given their approval; this, though, could be described as forced cooperation (Lofman et al. 2004; Meyer 1993).

It is good practice to provide the co-researchers with an information leaflet describing the clinical action research process and the nature of informed consent, anonymity, confidentiality and the right to withdraw from the project. A consent to participate form should also be provided. During the lifespan of an action research study other staff, including newly appointed staff, may wish to join the project. The ethics committee needs to be advised that the same informed consent process will be implemented. Bellman (2003), at a preliminary meeting, received signed consent forms from each of the co-researchers. The co-researchers also had the option of completing a short anonymous questionnaire to gauge their initial reactions. Questions included:

What are your expectations of the action research study? How do you feel about keeping a reflective journal?

According to Badger (2000), the very nature of interdisciplinary work in healthcare means that changing one profession's way of working affects others. Consequently, attempting to gain informed consent could result in resistance to change. This happened in a study in a surgical ward to implement patient self-medication, patient-controlled analgesia and operation information leaflets (Bellman 2003). One of the consultant surgeons did not wish his patients to participate in the study and so:

> We did not use his patients for the first phase of the study. In change theory terms (Rogers 1995) this surgeon was a 'late majority adopter'. When latterly he heard from his medical colleagues about the changes and developments taking place, he then requested that his patients should also be included in the study. (Bellman 2003: 70)

The cautions regarding informed consent for patients and carers include their ability to understand the information sufficiently to give their informed consent. A lack of understanding may indicate that the information is not precise enough (Lofman et al. 2004) or that the information needs to be presented in a more user-friendly way. The Gobbledygook Test is a useful tool for determining readability for different audiences (Oxford University Press 2010; see Box 7.2).

Box 7.2

A tool for determining readability of written material for adults (Oxford University Press 2010)

The gobbledygook test

This test measures the approximate level of difficulty of a piece of writing. It is a rough measure because it deals only with word length and sentence length. Many other variables, such as sentence structure and size of print, help to make reading easy or difficult. Never write just to please the test: a low score does not guarantee simplicity or clarity. Follow the instructions to work out the level of difficulty of the text, remembering that numbers and symbols are counted as short words, hyphenated words are counted as two words, and a syllable, for the purpose of the test, is a vowel sound. So *advised* is two syllables, *applying* is three.

Instructions	Sample A	Sample B	Sample C
1 Count a 100-word sample.			
2 Count the number of complete sentences in the Sample A column.			
3 Count the total number of words in all the complete sentences and note it in the sample A column.			
4 Find the average sentence length by dividing the answer for instruction 3 by the answer for instruction 2.			
5 Count the number of words of three or more syllables in the full 100 words. This gives the percentage of long words in the sample.			
6 Add the answers for instructions 4 and 5. This gives the test score for the sample.			
7 Repeat with two more samples, B and C.			
8 Add the three test scores. Test scores A + B + C =			

9 Divide by three to get a final average score. Average of A, B & C =			
10 Compare your score with the results below. (The lower the score, the more comprehensible the material is likely to be.)			

Woman Magazine	25
Sun newspaper	26
Daily Mirror	28
Daily Express	29
Daily Mail	31
Morning Star	34
Daily Telegraph	34
The Times	36
The Guardian	39
'Cars' (Office of Fair Trading leaflet)	40
Notes to British Visitor's Passport Application Form	45
Standard letter (Dept. of Employment)	49
'Conditions of Use' (Application for an Access credit card)	49

(The calculations on newspapers were made on 14 July 1980.)

* Adapted from R. Gunning's *FOG* (frequency of gobbledygook) formula. The formula is considered best for testing material for adult readers.

* The Gobbledygook Test is reprinted with the permission of the Plain English Campaign and the National Consumer Council.

Developing the research proposal and the content and language of the consent forms is a collaborative process (Brydon-Miller and Greenwood 2006). In the study by Bellman and Corrigan (2010), the co-researchers' research activities included:

- co-writing and submitting the internet research information system form for ethical approval;
- designing patient and staff consent forms and participant information forms.

• • • REFLECTIVE ACTIVITY 7.2 • • •

Use the Gobbledygook Test, Box 7.2, to determine the readability of the information that you and co-researchers have compiled for research participants and stakeholders.

Confidentiality and anonymity

In her research article, Spalding (2009) describes complying with the local research ethics committee's request to preserve participants' identities, and Waterman et al. (2005) state that participants were also assured that data would be anonymised and confidentiality maintained. According to Street (2008), constant vigilance is required to ensure that the anonymity of participants is not compromised within the reporting and dissemination of research findings. Yet, given the political nature of action research, it is difficult to guarantee confidentiality and anonymity (Williamson and Prosser 2002). No doubt others in the same organisation will know who participated. Also, while the guarantee of anonymity may protect participants from negative consequences, it also excludes them from public ownership of the data and recognition of their input into its use (AARE 2005). To resolve partly the ethical challenges of confidentiality and anonymity, participants need to feel that they have ownership of the data and feel able to control how the findings are more widely disseminated (Meyer 2000). Badger (2000) also suggests encouraging the co-researchers to scrutinise the research report and for the action researcher to maintain continuous feedback to participants. It may be difficult to disguise data or individuals in specific roles (Lathlean 1996), so there is a need to negotiate rules of confidentiality which are acceptable to all participants and for which all agree to accept responsibility (Winter and Munn-Giddings 2001). However, Hockley (2006: 100), in her study, cautions:

> Although I ensured that all identity of individual comments was avoided when feeding back data, I was not confident that all staff in the nursing home, the majority of whom were not used to participating in research, took on this responsibility. At one point in the study, I realised that much of what was being said in the collaborative learning group work was being reported back to management. This had a detrimental effect on the relationships between staff and the management of the nursing home. In trying to address this breach of confidentiality with management, it was obvious that management felt otherwise. Staff were remarkably tolerant of the situation but confidentiality had been breached and I felt very responsible.

All findings should be shared with participants to allow them to comment critically on whether they feel their views have been represented adequately and for them to check that they are happy for the material to be shared with a wider audience (Meyer 2010). Co-researchers may in fact choose to forego anonymity. With local and national dissemination of their project, the co-researchers may wish to be acknowledged for their contribution to enhancing the quality of patient care and may also choose to co-author the research project, co-publish a journal article and co-present the project at a research conference. Some co-researchers may also choose to write up their involvement for academic accreditation (for example, in Bellman et al. 2003).

Honesty and integrity

Conventional researchers have a duty to be honest in their explanations to participants; in action research this principle is absolute for co-researcher participation (Winter and Munn-Giddings 2001). It is important for the action researcher to state at the outset that they will not have all the answers and that the research process is a learning process for all involved. A communication strategy, developed with the co-researchers, ensures that the work of the project remains 'visible' to all participants and that discussions are fully documented (Winter and Munn-Giddings 2001). In the project undertaken by Bellman and Corrigan (2010), one way of ensuring high visibility and documentation was to audio-tape each co-researcher meeting. Each tape was then transcribed and the transcript emailed to each of the co-researchers for review. The Consultant Nurse co-researcher also produced a minuted version for discussion at follow-up meetings.

The need for personal truth and integrity is subsumed within the commitment by Brydon-Miller and Greenwood (2006: 126):

> We must continually challenge ourselves and one another to take responsibility for ensuring that our projects do real good for real people; that the claim to serve as agents of change is not an empty one. And we must resist complacency and a conviction of our own moral superiority by continually revisiting the issue of research ethics in both our teaching and our practice.

Ethical decision making in action research can include whether to undertake more than one patient-centred change. Elliott (1991) explains that an action research study is set up to deal with one issue, and therefore one change at a time should be planned, implemented and evaluated. However, like Bellman (2003), Spalding (2009) found that the clinical team she was facilitating were in receipt of a lot of data and wanted to plan multiple improvements:

> I did not deem it appropriate, or ethical, to delay suggested simultaneous improvements. (Spalding 2009: 136)

Withdrawing from the project

Respecting the right to withdraw from the study is a most important consideration for researchers on the road to equal relationships and interaction (Lofman et al. 2004). However, although a consent form clearly states the option to withdraw from the study at any time, this is a controversial issue in action research studies. Indeed, withdrawal may even jeopardise a whole project. Nevertheless the action researcher must respect a co-researcher's right to withdraw, as Hockley (2006: 98) demonstrates:

> It was in many ways difficult for staff not to take part (Kelly and Simpson 2001), especially when an action cycle became part of the development of practice in the nursing home. One person, however, requested formally to come out of the study during the facilitation phase.

The reason for withdrawal should be documented but may not always be evident. One reason for withdrawal could be when a co-researcher believes that they are making less of a contribution than their colleagues. Co-researchers usually participate to the best of their ability and all contributions are valued. However, the more extrovert co-researcher may appear to contribute more. Yet, a reflexive account reveals:

> No pressure was placed on the quiet co-researchers to speak. Yet, when they did speak it was powerful and significant as they reflected ideas that no one else had voiced. (Bellman 2003: 237)

It is important to recognise that pressure from within the group, or a perceived negative perception of them by a senior colleague/manager, may also make it seem difficult to withdraw. Sometimes a prolonged relationship between the action researcher and co-researchers can produce a felt obligation to help the researcher to 'succeed' (Trondsen and Sandaunet 2009). The action researcher should anticipate as many of these tensions as possible, although it may not be possible to identify them all (Streubert Speziale and Carpenter 2007).

The withdrawal of the action researcher either during a project or from an unfinished one could also present an ethical dilemma. Smith et al. (2009: 18) contemplated:

> Is it worth attempting to facilitate a change in practice when it is reasonably foreseeable that factors outside the control of the facilitators may inhibit the sustainability of the change?

Because of the challenges associated with ethical approval and the demands on staff in practice and academic settings, there is often slippage of the timeline. Harrison and Brandling (2010) found that because of the practical and ethical expectations of research within the National Health Service (NHS) they were obliged to identify and adhere to specific research milestones, in particular regarding data collection, analysis and writing up. Despite the authors' intentions and hopes, the project did not conclude with a defined set of practice changes. Fortunately for the co-researchers and patients, one of the co-facilitators was able to remain actively involved to address the long-term issues raised by the project.

• • • REFLECTIVE ACTIVITY 7.3 • • •

The ethical considerations in Box 7.3 were identified from an action research project (Lofman et al. 2004). In your project, how will you address informed consent, confidentiality and anonymity, protection from harm, potential exploitation and the role of the action researcher?

Box 7.3

Ethical considerations (Lofman et al. 2004)

Informed consent

- Informing patients about the research
- Point of times for giving information
- Right to withdraw
- Giving of consent
- Consent to the unknown
- Having 'joiners' in the research
- Getting the consent of 'joiners'

Confidentiality and anonymity

- Protection of identity
- Identification of a specific role
- Confidentiality of interviews

Protecting an individual from harm

- Intrusion into the lives of participants
- Value of the change
- Confrontation between the 'protector' and the 'protected'

The role of the action researcher

- Involvement of the researcher
- Unequal relationship
- Patronising of participants
- Unequal balance of power

Exploitation

- The ownership of the research
- Tension between initiator and participants
- Owning the outcomes
- Lack of support from authority
- Feeling of ownership and control

Research approval

The body which coordinates NHS research in the UK is called the NHS Research Ethics Service (NRES, see http: //www.nres.npsa.nhs.uk/). NRES has a dual mission:

- to protect the rights, safety, dignity and well-being of research participants;
- to facilitate and promote ethical research that is of potential benefit to participants, science and society.

All studies seeking to recruit participants who are staff or patients of the NHS must be approved through this service within IRAS, the Integrated Research Application System. IRAS is a single online system for applying for permissions and approvals for health and social care/community research in the UK. This involves a lengthy online application process. However, the Government continues to advocate simpler regulation of health research and to seek better ways to streamline the process.

In addition to approval from an ethics committee, Research Governance approval is also required. Research Governance frameworks are recognised internationally and are in place to ensure that the public can have confidence in, and benefit from, quality research in health and social care. The framework provides a context for the encouragement of creative and innovative research and for the effective transfer of learning, technology and best practice to improve care (Department of Health 2005: 3). The Research Governance Coordinator for the NHS Trust should be contacted to support the approval process for your research project.

Research ethics committees

Ethics committees are very familiar with traditional research approaches, particularly positivist research where the hypotheses, methodologies and anticipated outcomes can be articulated in advance. The approval or rejection of these projects is usually undertaken in a straightforward manner.

Difficulties can arise when members of ethics committees who have a limited or lack of understanding are confronted with new paradigm research proposals, even though democratic collaboration, co-generation of knowledge and a commitment to the democratisation of human situations are the major guidelines that action research follows (Brydon-Miller and Greenwood 2006). As Johnson (1997) previously identified, there is still a need for ethics committees and supervisory bodies for research to adopt a more facilitative approach to action research.

An ethics committee's limited understanding of action research requires the researcher to demonstrate that the methodology holds out more important guarantees for the ethical treatment of human subjects than does conventional research as it:

- is built on voluntary partnership between a researcher and local stakeholders who form a collaborative team that determines the subject and methods of the work

and they also:

- learn and apply the methods together;
- analyse the outcomes;
- design and implement the actions arising from the research process (Brydon-Miller and Greenwood 2006).

Understanding the needs of the ethics committee in regard to the nature and conduct of an action research project is sound preparation. Contacting the Chair of the Local Research Ethics Committee to review the proposal is recommended. For Waterman et al. (2005), the Chair's response was that there were no ethical objections to the project and that it need not be submitted formally for approval. However, for many action researchers there is still a continuing need to remind ethics committees that the methodology is a bona fide approach to research, and even then some members are simply mystified (Storch, personal communication 28/6/2010). The review and approval process for Storch et al. (2009) is depicted in Box 7.4. The process was seen as providing 'teachable moments' while obtaining approval.

Box 7.4

The ethical review and approval process for Storch et al. (2009)

1. Introduce the proposal overall and (obtain permission to) proceed to invite potential participants through group meetings or in whatever way works for the proposed research. Ethical approval is then given once people are recruited and have begun to be involved in determining the goals of the project.
2. An Amendment is submitted outlining the modified proposal as a function of research participants' input.
3. As the research proceeds and further modifications are made, amendments are submitted regularly and information provided regarding how the project is unfolding.
4. Finally, a completion report is submitted and that too is teachable time for outlining how this particular project unfolded.

Action researchers should realistically anticipate some delay in receiving approval for their project from an ethics committee and this should be reflected in the project timeline. From personal experience, an average delay of up to three months is anticipated. However, for Titchen and Manley (2006) the ethical committee hurdles were awesome. It was necessary to develop research protocols for tools (with participants) for multi-centred research ethics proposals which the authors stated would normally have been part of everyday practice. Crowley and Davis (2008) came to realise that research ethics committees do provide a valuable function, even though their mental health study, which focused on user- and carer-led practice development, was delayed for two years.

••• REFLEXIVE ACTIVITY 7.4 •••

Read the ethical and legal challenge for Crowley and Davis (Box 7.5) regarding carer involvement in research and consider how you would address the issue raised by the ethics committee.

Box 7.5

An ethical and legal challenge regarding carer involvement in research (Crowley and Davis 2008)

The research project has its origins in a depot medication clinic of a Community Mental Health Team (CMHT) in south London. A user receiving her three-weekly depot injection asked the community mental health nurse who was administering the injection whether there were any obstacles preventing her husband from giving her the depot injection. The service user wanted her husband to administer the depot injection every three weeks. However, since this practice intervention was not driven by local or national policies, was not research-based, and represented a potentially significant sea-change in clinical practice, culture and role, six months would elapse before it was seriously considered at a senior level within the team.

There is a growth, both nationally and internationally, of policies that promote user participation within health care (Nolan 2005). The rising number of patients with enduring mental health problems living in the community has led to providers of mental health services facing increasing pressure to meet their needs and the needs of those supporting them. The Trust's research and development (R&D) department supported an application to a Local NHS Research Ethics Committee (LREC). The application stated that the aims of the research study were:

- to explore the elements of risk management involved in enabling carers (supportive persons) to give depot injections;
- to develop a training package that may be useful for others to use should such a request be made;

- to establish whether enabling supportive persons to give depot injections would have an effect on the relationship between the user (recipient of the medication) and the supportive person (giver of medication).

Within the NHS, Research Ethics Committees (RECs) are responsible for ensuring all research projects comply with ethical frameworks, such as the Helsinki Declaration. Since seeking their opinion and review is mandatory for all NHS-based research, they have a secondary function in forcing researchers to think clearly and in detail about the ethical dimensions of their research. General discussion with the REC was unfavourable given that a possible scenario had not been considered within the application. The scenario was as follows:

- Nurse A, carer B and user C have been recruited to the research project.
- Nurse A teaches carer B to give user C a depot injection.
- What would happen if carer B has an 'off day' and makes an error or injured client C, and this arose not from a skills or knowledge deficit but rather accidentally or by chance?

The question raised by the LREC was therefore whether user C would be covered by existing NHS liability cover. This question could not be answered and the outcome of the LREC review was that this would need to be clarified before any favourable opinion could be offered.

Although the ethics committee provided supportive encouragement, clarifying the query they posed led to a two-year journey involving the local NHS Trust, the Trust's Legal Department, the Royal College of Nursing's Legal Department, the Nursing and Midwifery Council (NMC), the National Health Service Litigation Authority (NHSLA), research supervisors and numerous others. The desire by Crowley and Davis (2008) to seek clarification was further nurtured by their knowledge of practice in other healthcare disciplines where relatives are routinely engaged in the delivery of medications by injections, for example in child care (Evans 1994), rheumatology care (Arthur et al. 1999), palliative care (Lee and Headland 2003) and endocrinology treatment (Bevan et al. 2007). Following discussion with practitioners within these groups, it became increasingly clear that the question of liability had not been answered or indeed actively considered. This important and interesting article (Crowley and Davis 2008) addressing a significant ethical and legal issue encompasses prevention of harm, carer indemnity and NHS Trust membership of liability to third parties' schemes. The actual and potential impact on the project from this experience is recorded in Box 7.6. However, this experience should not deter future research with both patients and carers. For example, Williamson (2007) congratulates Glasson et al. (2006) on involving older participants, including those with conditions such as dementia, in their action research study.

Box 7.6

The impact on the study from the prolonged delay for approval by the ethics committee (actual and potential) (Crowley and Davis 2008)

- Shortened time-span for data collection, analysis and dissemination.
- Potential participants are lost to recruitment.
- Clinical team research-mindedness can decrease due to perceived complexity of obtaining NHS-based research approval.
- Study fatigue can set in for the action researcher and others.
- Interested and supportive managers and key staff may move on during a long approval process.
- Renegotiation of access to research sample may be required.
- Re-establishing negotiations and relationships with key personnel may be necessary.
- Changes to the Local Research Ethics Committee (LREC) system of online application required that a new application had to be formulated and submitted.

> 'It was very tempting to abandon the entire project but given the time invested and also the previously unconsidered clinical implications, it was felt that indemnity clarification was imperative. Also, it was considered inevitable that other clinicians working in a similar area would eventually encounter the same issues and, additionally, given that public money is involved, it made sense to continue.'

It is always advisable to attend the ethics committee meeting to clarify information and respond to queries. This may also result in lessening any delay in commencing the project. Any initial groundwork with the co-researchers that you have been able to undertake will be worthwhile, for example, informal discussion with colleagues/potential co-researchers of the methodology, and the nature of informed consent and anonymity and confidentiality, potential risks (if known), plus having the right to withdraw from the project at any time. Outright ethical approval may be granted but most researchers (whatever their chosen methodology) are often asked to provide further information or clarification.

Some action research studies, as stated, may require further ethical approval. This could sometimes be problematic, as Brydon-Miller and Greenwood (2006) recognise that sometimes action research can move very quickly and waiting for permission to continue could make it impossible for groups to act spontaneously or to reach a decision to engage in some immediate action. Titchen and Manley (2006) consider that practitioner-researchers need to have available to them research-based protocols that they can use to investigate their own practice, that are evidence based, and that do not require repeated ethical approval. Over-cautious ethics committees are taken to task by Brydon-Miller and Greenwood (2006: 122):

Efforts to minimise the likelihood of harm to human subjects by severely limiting the kinds of research that can be done, the questions that can be asked, and the types of individuals involved in the research, can, while providing protection, at the same time have the effect of making social research largely impotent in terms of addressing issues of real importance.

Summary

This chapter has demonstrated the need to adhere to the ethical principles of mutual respect, trustworthiness and transparency, fairness, informed consent, reciprocity (in terms of shared goals, dedication, responsibility, time and effort), and equal voice and full disclosures (Bastida et al. 2010). The action researcher needs to try to anticipate as many ethical issues as possible. Prerequisites for the researcher are to have a mindset of time, patience and endurance (Crowley and Davis 2008) and to clearly distinguish between coercion and a shared interest in promoting change and generating new knowledge (Brydon-Miller and Greenwood 2006).

It is anticipated that with the increase in action research proposals ethics committees will become more aware and appreciative of the methodology. Despite careful and considered planning, ethical issues can and do arise, particularly in regard to user and carer involvement in research. Taking a proactive approach in understanding the needs of ethics committees is highly recommended. For colleagues studying for a higher degree, finding a research supervisor who has both theoretical knowledge and practical expertise in doing action research is a priority.

Further reading

Long, T and Johnson, M (2007) *Research ethics in the real world: Issues and solutions for health and social care*. Oxford: Churchill Livingstone/Elsevier.

Royal College of Nursing (RCN) (2007) *User involvement in research by nurses: RCN guidance*. London: Royal College of Nursing.

Useful resources

National Research Ethics Service (NRES): www.nres.npsa.nhs.uk.

NHS Trusts' Research and Development departments may also have a research design support facility, will usually provide expertise regarding the IRAS submission, and possibly advise on funding sources.

Universities: Apart from programmes and modules for students to learn about research ethics, students at universities will be allocated an academic supervisor and often more than one so that different perspectives on the research project can be covered. This may take the form of one supervisor having an interest in the methodology to be used and one having an interest in the subject or field of study.

Generally students undertaking clinical action research projects for academic qualifications will need to get ethical approval through the university's ethics committee. Students will also require approval through IRAS and research governance approval from the NHS Trust or local authority bodies.

References

AARE (2005) Annotated Bibliography – Ethics in Educational Research. AARE the association for active educational researchers. http://www.aare.edu.au/ethics/aareethc.htm.

Arthur, A, Klinkhoff, A and Teufel, A (1999) Safety of self-injection of gold and methotrexate. *The Journal of Rheumatology*, 26: 302–305.

Badger, TG (2000) Action research, change and methodological rigour. *Journal of Nursing Management* 8: 201–207.

Bastida, E M, Tung-Sung, Tseng, McKeever, C and Jack Jr, L (2010) Ethics and community-based participatory research: Perspectives from the field. *Health Promotion Practice* 11(1): 16–20. DOI: 10.1177/1524839909352841 2010.

Bellman, L (1996) Changing nursing practice through reflection on the Roper, Logan and Tierney model: The enhancement approach to action research. *Journal of Advanced Nursing* 24(1): 129–138.

Bellman, L (2001) Courage, faith and chocolate cake: Requisites for exploring professionalism in action. *Educational Action Research* 9(2): 225–242. DOI: 10.1080/09650790100200147.

Bellman, L (2003) *Nurse-led change and development in clinical practice.* Nursing Research Series. London: Wiley-Blackwell.

Bellman L, Bywood C, & Dale S. (2003) Advancing working and learning through critical action research: creativity and constraints. *Nurse Education in Practice*, 3 (4): 186–194.

Bellman, L and Corrigan, P (2010) Using action research to develop a thoracic support nurse role to enhance quality of care. *Nursing Times* 106(22) (8–14 June): 18–21.

Bevan, J S, Newell-Price, J, Wass, J A H, Atkin, S L, Bouloux, P M, Chapman, J, Davis, J R E, Howlett, T A, Randeva, H S, Stewart, P M and Viswanath, A (2007) Home administration of lanreotide Autogel® by patients with acromegaly, or their partners, is safe and effective. *Clinical Endocrinology* 68(3): 343–349.

Brydon-Miller, M and Greenwood, D (2006) A re-examination of the relationship between action research and human subjects review processes. *Action Research* 4(1): 117–128.

Coghlan, D and Brannick, T (2010) *Doing action research in your own organisation* (3rd edition). London: Sage.

Crowley, J and Davis, A (2008) A researcher's journey for clarity: Clarifying liability and indemnity issues where carers take on a role in medicines management. *Journal of Psychiatric and Mental Health Nursing* 15: 717–721.

Department of Health (2005) *Research governance framework for health and social care* (2nd edition). London: Department of Health. Available online at: www.dh.gov.uk (last accessed 1/9/2010).

Elliott, J (1991) *Action research for educational change*. Milton Keynes/Buckingham: Open University Press.

Evans, M A (1994) An investigation into the feasibility of parental participation in the nursing care of their children. *Journal of Advanced Nursing* 20: 477–482.

French, J R P and Raven, B (1959) The bases of social power. In D Cartwright and A Zander (eds), *Group dynamics: Research and theory*. New York: Harper & Row.

Glasson, J, Chang, E, Chenoweth, L, Hancock, K, Hall, T and Hill-Murray, F (2006) Evaluation of a model of nursing care for older patients using participatory action research in an acute medical ward. *Journal of Clinical Nursing* 15(5): 588–598. DOI: 10.1111/j.1365-2702.2006.01371.x.

Harrison, A and Bradling, J (2010) Using action research to address the mental health needs of older people: A reflection and discussion of real-world problems. *Educational Action Research* 18(2): 255–272.DOI: 10.1080/09650791003741772.

Hart, E and Bond, M (1995) *Action research for health and social care: A guide to practice*. Buckingham: Open University Press.

Hockley, J (2006) Developing high quality end-of-life care in nursing homes an action research study. PhD thesis, University of Edinburgh and Steinberg Collection, RCN.

Hope, K (1998) Starting out with action research. *Nurse Researcher* 6: 16–26.

Jinks, A M and Chalder, G (2007) Consensus and diversity: An action research study designed to analyse the roles of a group of mental health consultant nurses. *Journal of Clinical Nursing* 16(7) (July): 1323–1332.

Johnson, M (1997) Observations on the neglected concept of intervention in nursing research. *Journal of Advanced Nursing* 25: 23–29.

Kelly, Dand Simpson, S (2001) Action research in action: Reflections on a project to introduce clinical practice facilitators to an acute hospital setting. *Journal of Advanced Nursing* 33: 652–659.

Lathlean J. (1996) Ethical dimensions in action research. In Nursing Research. An Ethical and Legal Appraisal, Chapter 3 (de Raeve L. ed.), Bailliere Tindall, London

Lee, L and Headland, C (2003) Administration of as required subcutaneous medications by lay carers: Developing a procedure and leaflet. *International Journal of Palliative Nursing* 9: 142–149.

Lofman, P, Pelkonen, M and Pietila, A (2004) Ethical issues in participatory action research. *Scandinavian Journal of Caring Sciences*, 18: 333–340.

Meyer, J (1993) New paradigm research in practice: The trials and tribulations of action research. *Journal of Advanced Nursing* 18: 1066–1072.

Meyer, J (2000) Evaluating action research. *Age and Aging* 29: 8–10.

Meyer, J (2010) Action research. In K Gerrish and A Lacey (eds), *The research process in nursing* (6th edition). Oxford: Wiley-Blackwell, Chapter 22.

Minkler, M, Fadem, P, Perry, M, Blum, K, Moore L and Rogers, J (2002) Ethical dilemmas in participatory action research: A case study from the disability community. *Health Education and Behaviour*, 29: 14–29.

Munhall, P L (2001) *Nursing research: A qualitative perspective* (3rd edition). Sudbury, MA: Jones and Barlett.

NMC (2008) *The code: Standards of conduct, performance and ethics for nurses and midwives*. London: Nursing and Midwifery Council. Available online at: www.nmc-uk.org/Nurses-and-midwives/The code/ (accessed 11/08/2010).

Nolan, M.R. (2005) Reconciling tensions between research, evidence-based practice and user participation: Time for nursing to take the lead. *International Journal of Nursing Studies* 42, 503-505.

Oxford University Press (2010) *The Gobbledygook Test*. Online resource centre, www.oup.com/uk/orc/bin/9780199212712/resources/gobble (accessed 01/09/2010).

Rogers, E M (1995) *Diffusion of innovations* (4th edition). New York: Free Press.

Smith, S, Lewis, P and Wilson, V (2009) A 'wee' problem: Using action research to facilitate a change in urine collection methods. *Neonatal, Paediatric and Child Health Nursing* 12(1): 15–19.

Spalding, N J (2009) Improving practice through involvement in action research. *International Journal of Therapy and Rehabilitation* 16(3): 130–138.

Storch, J, Rodney, P, Pauly, B, Fulton, T R, Stevenson, L, Newton, L and Makaroff, K S (2009) Enhancing ethical climates in nursing work environments. *Canadian Nurse* 105(3): 20–25.

Street, A (2008) An action research inquiry exploring the transfer of pain knowledge from a continuing education course into practice. PhD thesis, University of Stirling. Available online at: http://hdl.handle.net/1893/474 and Steinberg collection, RCN.

Streubert Speziale, H J and Carpenter, D R (2007) *Qualitative research in nursing: Advancing the humanistic imperative*. London: Lippincott Williams and Wilkins.

Titchen, A and Manley, K (2006) Spiralling towards transformational action research: Philosophical and practical journeys. *Educational Action Research* 14(3): 333–356.

Trondsen, M and Sandaunet, A (2009) The dual role of the action researcher. *Evaluation and Program Planning* 32: 13–20.

Waterman, H, Harker, R, MacDonald, H, McLaughlan, R and Waterman, C (2005) Advancing ophthalmic nursing practice through action research. *Journal of Advanced Nursing* 52(3): 281–290.

Williamson, G and Prosser, S (2002) Action research, politics, ethics and participation. *Journal of Advanced Nursing* 40(5): 587–593.

Williamson, T (2007) Commentary on Glasson J, Chang E, Chenoweth L, Hancock K, Hall, T and Hill-Murray F (2006) Evaluation of a model of nursing care for older patients using participatory action research in an acute medical ward. *Journal of Clinical Nursing* 15, 588–598. *Journal of Clinical Nursing* 16(10): 1981–1982.

Winter, R and Munn-Giddings, C (eds) (2001) *A handbook for action research in health and social care*. London: Routledge.

SECTION 4

DISSEMINATING AND EVALUATING CLINICAL ACTION RESEARCH PROJECTS

8

WRITING CLINICAL ACTION RESEARCH STUDIES

Loretta Bellman, Jonathan Webster and Graham R Williamson

The increasing number of action research studies being undertaken reinforces the need for more accounts on ways in which to write them. The focus of this chapter is what to write, and how to convey clinical action research projects in different ways. General guidance for writing action research projects is now included in some action research texts. While considering the general guidance, what else you write depends very much on the type of account you wish to produce, ranging from a thesis, internal report, to a topical article in a professional journal.

Chapter objectives

The objectives of the chapter are to:

- highlight key areas to address in the writing of clinical action research studies;
- differentiate between internal report writing, writing for a higher degree and writing articles for publication in academic and peer-reviewed 'popular' journals;
- consider the challenges, criticism and creativity that surrounds the writing of clinical action research projects.

The aim of writing is to convey the process, outcomes and key messages of an action research project in appropriate ways to meet the needs of the readership. The readership may include clinical colleagues, senior health service managers, service users and carers, students, doctoral examiners and academic colleagues.

Key areas to address

Unless you have chosen to write a journal article which focuses on a specific aspect of action research (for example, ethical considerations) most clinical action research accounts will need to include, to a greater or lesser extent:

a how the project originally evolved and a description of the political context;
b a critique of action research literature and justification for the chosen methodology;
c your role and whether you consider yourself to be an insider or outsider action researcher or both (see Chapter 4);
d how the clinical context for the project was selected;
e how the co-researchers became involved, a description of their roles and the clinical context;
f how you *facilitated* the *collaborative* process, including –

1. agreeing the research questions or objectives
2. agreeing research participants
3. reaching a consensus on the focus of change and project timeline
4. leading the ethical research process and any issues that arose
5. action planning
6. agreeing/accessing/devising data collection methods
7. undertaking data collection
8. undertaking the data analysis process and reaching consensus regarding the resultant direction of the project
9. stating how changes were introduced and evaluated
10. dealing with problems and organisational challenges, e.g. resistance to change, role conflict, disempowering processes
11. detailing process and outcome evaluation with the co-researchers.

g how you have ensured rigour (Chapter 2);
h key outcomes of the project to date and the next steps, or an open-ended account. In some respects an action research study does not simply end (Winter and Munn-Giddings 2001);
i learning outcomes from participation in the study through action researcher reflexivity and co-researcher feedback/outcome evaluation.

Writing internal reports

The purpose of an internal report is to effectively communicate the processes and outcomes of a clinical action research study to members of the organisation in which it was conducted. Most healthcare and academic staff carry heavy workloads so a well-written, succinct, internal report is to be welcomed. Stringer (2007: 169) cautions that because of the status enjoyed by science in the modern world, many organisations, including health institutions, universities and Government departments, try to replicate the formats of experimental scientific research in their reporting procedures. The challenge for the action researcher is therefore to construct an internal report that is true to the principles of action research (as above) and is both understandable and has the required impact for bureaucratic, academic, technical and non-technical audiences. Also, if financial support has been received for all or part of the project, then reports are required by the funder, often at different stages of the project, as well as a final report.

There is a wealth of literature regarding how to write up an action research study for a higher degree (see below). However, action research texts also need to incorporate internal report writing. This is a missed opportunity which needs to be rectified. The professional and political importance of disseminating practitioner-led, patient-centred research within healthcare organisations via internal reporting should not be underestimated.

• • • REFLECTIVE ACTIVITY 8.1 • • •

Whether you were able to complete your project, have had to leave it open-ended (h above), or are at a certain phase of the research: what do you consider are the benefits of producing an internal report of your project for the health care organisation in which you work?

For the benefit of service users, staff and the whole organisation, there is a professional responsibility to share the work you are doing, which will include both positive outcomes as well as f10 above. Nurses and midwives have a responsibility to make a difference to the quality of patient care by raising the profile of their research and development activity (McCance et al. 2006). Clinical and academic colleagues will be able to assess the transferability of your work, as well as be informed of the action research process (a–i above). Political benefits for the NHS Trust Board/senior managers include the implementation of healthcare policy, for example the *High Quality of Care For All* report (Darzi 2008) and patient involvement (Department of Health 2010). The report may also help to strengthen a two-way partnership of hospital and university support for practitioner-research in clinical practice.

You will need to resolve the controversial ethical dilemma as to whether the co-researchers and participants can be identified in the report by seeking their consent (see also Chapter 7). The co-researchers may choose to co-author the report. Personal profiles and careers may be enhanced by facilitating and participating in the project, and you, the co-researchers and colleagues in the clinical area where change and innovation have taken place will be future resources within the organisation and beyond (for example, see Box 8.1). Internal reports may be placed on the organisation's intranet and also be disseminated further afield. Positive consequences may result, including being asked to present your work both within the organisation and to external audiences (see also Chapter 9).

Box 8.1

Recognition of co-researchers as a very good resource for patients and staff (Bellman 2003: 138)

Manager evaluation interview

> This ward is now used as a resource. The rest of the hospital are very interested in what has been happening on patient self-medication now it is up and running and with PCA (patient controlled analgesia) too. When someone phones me to say they have a patient returned from theatre with PCA, who wasn't prepared, and what should they do, I tell them to contact a member of ward A. I've told them how good, very good, they are at educating both patients and staff.

••• REFLECTIVE ACTIVITY 8.2 •••

What should you and the co-researchers consider before starting to produce an internal report?

Box 8.2 lists key questions to consider when preparing to write an internal report. According to Gray (2009: 530), the questions that busy readers will ask themselves are:

> Does the title sound relevant or interesting to me?
>
> Do the contents of the report actually match the title?
>
> How long is the report – what is my investment of time going to be and is it worthwhile?
>
> How well presented is the report – how confident am I in the abilities of the writer?

Box 8.2

Questions to consider for internal reports

- Who may wish to read the report?
- Who wishes to be involved in writing the report? How will we share the input?
- What is the required timeline?
- How do we write a report that will be read?
- How politically sensitive is the information to be reported?
- How long should the report be?
- What structure is required?
- Is the report well presented and how do we know if it is user-friendly?
- When is the best time to distribute the report?
- How will the report be disseminated?
- What will be the anticipated impact of the report on different stakeholders?
- How will feedback from stakeholders be addressed?

Further advice is provided by Winter and Munn-Giddings (2001: 243) regarding what makes a piece of writing persuasive. The authors suggest that the writing needs to make readers feel that they are in 'safe hands', that they can trust you, and that you need to keep them sufficiently interested to follow your argument.

The internal report is for a mixed audience. Readers of the report are all the project participants plus the stakeholders. All readers are encompassed into two types: those who commissioned or who are expecting to read the report, and those who are not expecting the report but who may, none the less, be interested in it (Gray 2009). You should assume that there will be many stakeholders in the organisation, possibly also in partner organisations. Stakeholders are often operational managers plus those in strategic management positions (clinical and academic), peers and professional clinical and academic colleagues within your own and partnership organisations, and any funders. Also, as the focus of a project will be service users/carers, they may wish to receive the report. Depending on the organisation in which you work, patient representatives may include Patient Governors and members of Patient Forums who will also be essential report recipients.

Winter and Munn-Giddings (2001: 242) suggest that it is most useful to imagine that you are writing for well-informed colleagues in the same area of practice. However, as identified above, you are in fact writing for a range of stakeholders. Consider including a Glossary in the report to define what may be unfamiliar terminology for readers.

As the project timeline is developed, you will need to determine co-researcher collaboration in report writing. Report writing is a skill that takes time to develop; a flexible timeline is often an inevitable consequence.

A number of drafts may be required before the final report is completed to everyone's satisfaction. Co-researchers' input may vary depending on their motivation and time, but ensure that all authors' names appear on the title page of the report. The report will be widely read if it contains relevant and useful new information which is clearly presented and signposted, and is easily accessible. However, all the implications of the project are not always appreciated or, indeed, how the report will eventually be received. It is recommended that you check the political sensitivity of the report by forwarding a final draft copy to the Chief Executive, Dean, or equivalent. You should state who the intended recipients will be, offer to provide further information in person, and invite feedback. In most instances there should be a favourable response to proceed.

The length of the report is an individual matter but must include points a–i in the above list in a succinct way. For the reader to have an overview of the project and to decide, from the structure of the report, whether to read further, the report has to have an Executive Summary (of one–two pages) (Box 8.3) and a list of the contents that are page numbered (Box 8.4). You can help the reader to appreciate your project by using clear sign-posting and the creative use of tables, boxes, diagrams, etc. Table 8.1 provides one way of presenting an action research study for an internal report.

Box 8.3

Executive summary for an action research internal report (Bellman and Wiseman 2010)

Executive summary

Nurses and midwives have a responsibility to make a difference to the quality of patient care by raising the profile of their research and development (R&D) activity (McCance et al. 2006). The aim of the three-phase study is to explore how nurses and midwives are able to both conduct and use research in practice for patient benefit. There is increasing recognition that strong leadership is required, both clinical and academic, to support research and development opportunities for nurses and midwives in NHS Trusts (Carter 2007; Jackson and Butterworth 2007). The focus of Phase 1 was to identify the drivers and barriers to using and doing nursing and midwifery research in clinical practice with key stakeholders in the Trust, higher education providers, and the Strategic Health Authority.

An action research methodology enabled three research facilitators: Principal Investigator (Senior Nurse R&D), an external researcher and a Clinical Research Nurse) to collaborate with five Consultant Nurses and the Consultant Midwife, called the co-researchers. Research methods included semi-structured interviews and focus groups. In total there were 73 participants in this exploratory phase of the study. A three-stage data analysis process enabled the explication of six key themes which encompass the participants' perspectives of current drivers and barriers to change:

- The struggle continues
- Focus of nursing research and development
- Academic input into practice-based research
- Support within the Trust
- Lacking visibility
- Moving Forward?

Key recommendations from Phase 1 are: (1) Both long-term strategic planning and operational development are required to enable a clinical-academic leadership infrastructure for nursing and midwifery R&D; (2) the R&D role of Consultant Nurses/Midwife, and Advanced Practitioner colleagues, requires organisational recognition and clinical-academic support and development.

The focus of Phase 2 of the study is to systematically explore with nurse leaders their research and development role, and how to enable both the use of research findings in practice and the conduct of research in clinical practice. Funding for the project has been provided by The Burdett Trust.

Box 8.4

Contents page of an action research report for an internal audience and for the funder (Bellman and Wiseman 2010)

CONTENTS **Page**

(Continued)

(Continued)

Appendices

Table 8.1 An overview of the action research process and methods used for an action research project

Overview of the Thoracic Support Nurse (TSN) role development project	
Action research process	**Research methods**
1 Role development – ongoing review How is the role to be developed? What are the barriers and drivers to role development?	• Audio-taped co-researcher review meetings/ focused group reflection • TSN clinical supervision sessions • TSN reflective journal • TSN daily activity sheet • Staff perceptions & expectations questionnaire
2 Action planning What has to be done to enable role development? How can the barriers be addressed?	• Audio-taped co-researcher review meetings • Action Plan Consensus
3 Role implementation – ongoing feedback How do staff perceive role development? What changes are being initiated to enhance the quality of care for thoracic patients? How can the role be supported and embedded?	• Audio-taped co-researcher process evaluation • TSN clinical supervision • TSN reflective journal • Electronic staff survey tool • Audio-taped staff focus groups
4 Establishing the role – process & outcome evaluation What are the strengths of the role? What changes have occurred for patients/the TSNs/the co-researchers as a direct result of the project? What have the co-researchers learnt from engaging in the research project?	• Patient evaluation questionnaire • Audio-taped Divisional Senior Nurse semi-structured interview • Audio-taped co-researcher critical reflexivity/ group process & outcome evaluations

It is essential to clearly represent participants' voices. Indeed, with qualitative data much of the report may be presented through the voices of the participants. As well as the use of appropriate quotations, other literary devices may be employed. Stringer (2007: 120) suggests a variety of ways to represent participants' experiences, new knowledge, understanding, and the pragmatic outcomes of the project. You will need to consider the appropriateness of using alternative literary devices, for example, poems, narratives, memoirs, photographs, artwork, etc., when producing an internal report for a bureaucratic organisation.

• • • REFLECTIVE ACTIVITY 8.3 • • •

What alternative literary devices could you use to represent aspects of your project?

According to Gray (2009: 533), it may be worthwhile noting problems encountered in undertaking the research, the false starts made and negative findings recorded, so that other researchers may learn from your experience. In an action research project, point f10 in the list above is a fundamental part of the change process. In an internal report, describing these challenges and the extent to which they were overcome is important information for all readers within the organisation. Of key importance are the outcomes of the project (examples of positive outcomes are to be found in Table 8.2). Recommendations should then flow logically from the evidence in the report and are usually presented in a concise format (as in the executive summary example shown in Box 8.3). To gauge understanding, you should provide drafts marked confidential so that trusted colleagues can give you constructive feedback. Also, to test the readability of the report for different audiences, the Gobbledegook Test can be useful (see Chapter 7, Box 7.2).

Once the report is completed you may wish to seek advice for an appropriate time to circulate it. Use mail whenever possible, and state that feedback will be welcomed, preferably within 4–6 weeks of receiving the report. Also, if there is an internal newsletter produced within your organisation, you may want to provide a user-friendly brief account, and/or publish the report on the intranet to provide further information and wide dissemination. Feedback from participants and stakeholders can be very enlightening (see Box 8.5). As with other action research processes, you should consider that writing an internal report and receiving feedback takes longer than anticipated and adjust the timeline accordingly.

Table 8.2 Outcomes of the action research study for patients, co-researchers, manager, action researcher, clinical area, Hospital Trust (Bellman 2003: 161)

Patients	Nurses (co-researchers)	Manager	Action researcher	Clinical area	Hospital Trust
Increased psychological and physical independence	More insight into nursing More questioning of the status quo	'Eye opener'	Realisation of personal ideals: Learning in clinical practice Shared knowledge Patient participation Nurse empowerment	Enhanced team cohesion	Resource area for other units
Feeling in control	Work collaboratively	Recognition of nurses' abilities	Work collaboratively	Group goal attainment	Published information booklets
Increased knowledge	Enhanced knowledge	Valuing nurses' ideas	Group reflection skills	Proactive innovative setting	Enhanced patient satisfaction
Felt nurses trusted them	Enhanced teaching skills	Empowering nurses	Insight into strengthening multi-professional collaboration	Motivated nurses	Enhanced quality of care
Reduced feelings of anxiety	Feelings of personal achievement Enhanced nurse/patient communication Increased self-confidence Motivated towards further study Feeling able to make changes Increased writing skills		Enhanced knowledge	Enhanced quality of care	Improved staff morale

Box 8.5

Types of feedback from participants and stakeholders

The responses provide an opportunity to appreciate:

- how favourably the report was received;
- whether recipients understood the key messages in the report;
- what clarification will be required;
- interest from colleagues for the positive outcomes of the project;
- the wider need for action research education and application;
- support to sustain the positive outcomes of the project;
- the impact of the report on the organisation to support strategic/culture change and development.

Writing for a higher degree

A doctoral thesis or Masters dissertation, while encompassing a–i in the 'Key areas to be addressed' section above, is very different from an organisational internal report (above). Writing up clinical action research studies at higher degree level for many is a time to reflect on a journey of development, learning, insight and understanding. Of paramount importance is the extent to which the change process has been achieved and has impacted on patient care/clinical practice.

According to McNiff and Whitehead (2009: 122), most higher education institutions stipulate the following criteria for research Masters dissertations:

- The work makes a claim to knowledge.
- The work demonstrates a critical engagement with the ideas in the literature.

For doctoral level study, the thesis is the pinnacle of many action researcher's hours of hard work and determination. The difference between Masters and doctoral research is that at Masters level there does not need to be an original claim to knowledge, whereas this must be demonstrated at doctoral level. At Masters level students must:

- Demonstrate the methodological rigour of the research undertaken
- Demonstrate engagement and critical critique of the literature within the field of study and
- Develop your own conceptual frameworks, drawing from the literature. (McNiff and Whitehead 2009: 123)

The need for rigour and critique leading to either an original claim of 'new knowledge' (doctoral level) or the testing of a claim against other people's ideas (Master level) are critical themes at both levels of study. In addition, translating knowledge and understanding for the clinical action researcher into practice is vital, the ultimate goal being to improve care for people accessing health services. Sharing learning, knowledge and understanding with others in a way that is enabling and meaningful to them will also be key.

Collating large amounts of data presented in different formats into a cohesive, academic piece of writing that truly reflects the authentic journey that the clinical action research will have been on (over a significant period of time) requires clear thinking and a systematic way of working. It requires processing and presenting potentially different methods of data collection into a coherent analysis, discussion and conclusion. It also requires time and the space to critique and critically reflect. The examiners will wish to see a systematic approach and aclear audit trail of how you and the co-researchers conducted the research process. In addition, at the doctoral level, examiners are looking for:

- Originality – the contribution to knowledge
- Critical engagement: with own learning (reflexive critique); contextual issues (**dialectic**al critique); with the appropriateness of the literature
- A text of 'outstanding' technical excellence that is worthy of a peer-reviewed publication. (McNiff and Whitehead 2009: 139)

Demonstrating engagement with scholarly/professional debate forms a crucial element of both dissertation and thesis presentation (UniSA 2010). We discuss how the concept of dialectics (McNiff and Whitehead 2009) is applied to action research in Chapters 1 and 2, and the central importance of reflexivity in Chapter 2. For example, in the research diaries of Williamson (2004), he makes explicit his thoughts and feelings concerning his project with student support staff at his university and local NHS Trusts. He found this approach beneficial because it added a level of understanding that was heightened because of the reflexivity it entailed. He argued:

> My proximity to the research is a source of strength, in the sense that it allows access to participants and to sources of data, but is a weakness if it drives my interpretation of events. (Williamson 2004: 92)

He used his diaries to lay bare his assumptions, record project events and uncover hidden meaning with his organisation. This reflexivity was important in guiding his thinking and linked to ongoing discussion with others in the research team.

In capturing the authenticity of their work at either Masters or doctoral level, clinical action researchers need to be ordered and able to present their research in a way that is universally acceptable (in achieving an academic award), while maintaining the truth behind their work. For some clinical action researchers this can pose a tension, if they are expected to conform to a traditional scientific method of presenting a dissertation or thesis in a format that is at 'odds' with the learning and creativity underpinning their research. Higgs and Titchen (2001: 5) identify that tensions can occur in professional practice and research between rational, intuitive and creative thinking and between art and science. They argue that by making sense and valuing these different elements that underpin personal knowledge, an attempt can be made to 'bridge' the theory–practice gap. As part of the evaluation of his doctoral action research study, Webster (2007) recognised the need to balance the use of artwork (drawings) and semi-structured interviews. Through negotiation with the doctoral supervisory team, he presented in his thesis artwork by participants alongside a thematic analysis of interviews. He stated:

> This level of creativity felt appropriate for the evaluation as a key intention of the programme of practice development was focussed on developing creativity in both professional practice with older people and thinking. (Webster, 2007: 89)

For any student undertaking either a Masters or doctoral pathway, negotiating complementary ways of writing up a project can be challenging. However, for doctoral students, this can be more critical (given the depth and scale of doctoral research) and highlights a simple message: choose your university and supervisors carefully and latterly identify an external examiner who, through their writing, you deem to be on your wave length! A university that places little value on action research, or supervisors who have little or no experience of action research as a methodology, may pose significant challenges to the clinical action researcher. Similarly, an external examiner who shares no common understanding or who has a totally opposing view may provide an unwelcome additional challenge after many years of hard work.

In her writing on 'discourse community', Lee (1998: 122) asserts the importance of acknowledging the audience and makes a case for the centrality of language in the process of research.The clinical action researcher therefore needs to be mindful of who their audience will be when writing up their study. Negotiation with the supervisory team, along with following the guidance published by the university on dissertation or thesis presentation, is crucial. Reading other action research studies at the university, Royal College of Nursing library etc. may also help the clinical action researcher shape and define their study when presenting it for examination. Peer support, including constructive criticism, can also be valuable in helping critical reflection, learning and development in how themes, discussions, arguments and conclusions are clearly constructed and subsequently presented.

• • • REFLECTIVE ACTIVITY 8.4 • • •

As you write up your thesis or dissertation:

- consider creative, complementary ways of writing up parts of your project;
- identify project-specific articles for publication;
- consider publishing an article to address the current gaps in the literature related to conducting clinical action research.

Writing articles for publication in academic and peer-reviewed 'popular' journals

A key question when deciding to write an article is: Where shall I publish my study? Action researchers and co-researchers need to decide which journal to target to publish their project. There are a number of distinctions to be drawn between academic and 'popular' journals. Practitioners are more likely to read 'popular' journals on a regular basis so this can be an effective way of disseminating patient-centred research projects. Indeed, the co-researchers in the study by Bellman and Corrigan (2010) specifically requested that the study be published in a popular journal.

• • • REFLECTIVE ACTIVITY 8.5 • • •

What are the key differences between academic and peer-reviewed 'popular' journals?

Academic journals appear to serve a largely academic audience; popular journals are more widely read but do not devote so many pages to research studies or expect so much detail from those they do publish. University academics are required to publish papers annually, are graded on their performance in periodic research assessment exercises and secure funding for their departments as a result. They are concerned with the international reputation of journals as well as their 'impact factors' (which measures how often papers in a journal are cited by others). While they too would wish their study to be read by clinical practitioners, for them, targeting the right journals can be a career-enhancing activity. Others wanting recognition for their work may be happy to aim at the popular journals, which are likely to be circulated more widely to practising nurses in one country rather than internationally, and as the popular journals have less stringent requirements and expectations, it is considered easier to get studies published in them.

Writing for publication in an academic journal requires a different process compared to internal report writing or to writing for a research degree. You will be restricted to a word count (as you are for the others), using a format that suits the journal, and applying the journal's house style for referencing, tables and figures. The most important piece of advice is to identify your journal before you start to write as this enables you to write to the particular style of your target journal. All journal websites will have detailed guidelines for authors, including how to write your article and how to submit it. There's little point writing an essay-type piece and then finding out that it needs a substantial re-write when you look at the journal's requirements. Make sure you use a referencing software program like EndNote or Reference Manager as they will allow you automatically to do your referencing in the journal's style, and alter it quickly and easily. It can be challenging to secure a publication in one of the international journals such as *Journal of Advanced Nursing, Journal of Research in Nursing* or *International Journal of Nursing Studies*, and if you want to aim for a high-status journal such as these you may need support from an experienced author. Your work will be peer reviewed and you will receive feedback, but you may have to allow up to several months for this. It is highly unusual (and you are to be congratulated) if your article gets accepted without any amendments to the original submission. Be prepared to do either major or minor corrections. Although rare, your work can also be rejected, in which case, target what may be, for you, a more suitable journal, but do not give up as rejection is the beginning of the next submission!

Generally, journals require research studies to be written in the traditional IMRAD format, which is Introduction, Methods, Results and Discussion (and usually with a conclusions section). You will also be required to produce a succinct abstract with the same structure/key words which describe the article, and to give a statement on the role of each author in the project and in the production of the manuscript. The title is also very important. It needs to 'catch the eye' of the potential reader and sound interesting enough for them to wish to read your article. Each of the sections is discussed below:

Introduction. This should set the scene, arguing why the research study was necessary in the context of previous literature, policy and local setting. In an action research study, these will all be important, but local context will be essential for readers trying to interpret what you have done, why you have done it, who was involved and what was achieved. The literature should be reviewed critically, with an eye on gaps and/or trends, and it should be clear how the literature and policy have informed your work. For example, perhaps a policy document or NICE guideline indicated a particular change to clinical practice and, while lots of randomised controlled trials indicated that the new practice was effective, implementation had been slow or ineffective. Your action research study would therefore be justified; it would be addressing a pressing clinical need, and would also be bound up with the local service context. Your introduction should also state your aims and objectives: what you were trying to do and how you intended to proceed. So, your aim is to implement change and your objectives include working in collaborationwith the multidisciplinary team to foster a sense of ownership in the new changes. A good action research article introduction will address points a, b and d in the 'Key areas to address' section (above).

Methods. Even though an action research study is radically different in philosophical approach from traditional research, such as randomised controlled trials (RCTs), it will still have methods of data collection and analysis and they must be described. It will be worth starting with a section on the methodology and principles of the action research approach that you used in your study, as this will set the scene and give the reader a sense of your intention for collaboration and participation. A diagram of the 'journey' will be useful, showing how you planned to move thorough the phases or cycles of inquiry. Next, discuss your data collection methods: Interviews? Focus groups? Surveys? Observations? How did you and the co-researchers collect data and how did you analyse it? Points e and f from 'Key areas to address' (above) will be covered in the Methods section.

You will be required to make some statement that ethical clearance has been given by relevant bodies. If you are working with NHS staff or patients, this will be the NHS Research Ethics Service and you will also need local research governance approval from each NHS Trust. Local Authorities and universities have separate arrangements.

Results. If possible, it is preferable to refer to these as 'findings' rather than 'results', as the latter can indicate what you get from experiments! In a traditional study such as an RCT, the results will be tables and statistical analysis, but this will be very different in an action research (AR) study. It may need to involve a timetable of meetings and how the project actually developed, in contrast to your plan. You should show how you actually went through your phases or cycles, what insights were gained and how they influenced the direction of your work and your thinking. In addition, you will need to give findings from your data collection methods. For example, if you used focus groups, what themes emerged and what interaction took place? You will need to use quotes to illustrate this. If you used a questionnaire survey at any point, what were the results of this? The results section will demonstrate point h from the 'Key areas to address' section (above).

Discussion. This is where you will pull it all together. What did the results mean? What changes were you able to affect (if any)? What new knowledge was accrued as a result of the project? How was collaboration fostered and with whom? Local project insights should be compared and contrasted with the literature on the issue, and this may include some papers that you cited in your introduction as well as others. This is how you locate your work in a wider context to show transferability to other settings (as it will not be generalisable in the strict quantitative sense). Remember to state explicitly the extent to which your aims and objectives were achieved, and refer to any problems you encountered. If your project was 'unsuccessful' in the sense that you did not affect change, it is unlikely that it was a failure: what new knowledge was gathered? What were the issues, challenges and obstacles you faced and how were they overcome (or not)? What can others learn about implementation and/or collaboration on this issue from the difficulties you experienced in attempting to change practice? In the discussion, you should cover points c, g and i from the 'Key areas to address' section (above).

Conclusions. This should provide a short synopsis of your work, identify gaps in knowledge where possible, and give recommendations for future research, education and practice issues. No new material should be introduced and this section should be relatively short.

Abstract. Write this last! You will not be able to write it until the rest of the paper is completed. Remember, it needs to be the length specified by the journal. If you are submitting it electronically, the box will stop you putting in too many words. The abstract is really important as it gives readers an idea of what the paper is about and whether or not they want to read it. It should be a succinct summary, probably structured using the IMRAD format, and needs to be clear and accessible.

Title. You may have a clear project title which you've been working with all the way through, which will then become the title of the article, but if not, it is feasible to leave naming your article until it is finished. The title should be like a newspaper headline in that it summarises what the project is about (although not the methods or findings) and gives readers an idea of what to expect. It is useful to say that it is a clinical action research study and include the field of study. It may be preferable not to overdo anything cryptic or 'humorous' in the title as you're aiming for a professional presentation of your project, but a catchy title can be informative.

Key words. How many of these are required will be specified by the journal. The importance of key words lies in making your article accessible to others via electronic database searches, which is how potential readers will access your work. Virtually everyone uses electronic database searching these days, and if they are not doing so, they will be unsystematic in their search and will be limited in what they find in their university or hospital library. Choosing your key words carefully ensures that your article is accessible to interested readers. Electronic submission systems will often ask you to suggest key words from a drop-down list and this ensures consistency.

Authorship. It used to be reasonably common for postgraduate students and junior staff in universities to 'gift' authorship to revered colleagues and professors in their departments. This process enabled them to be seen as part of an important network, and giving these people publications that they had not worked on contributed to their publication rates. More recently, this gifted authorship has been reduced by journals requiring a list of 'who did what' in their articles, specifically who was responsible for study design, data collection and analysis, and manuscript preparation. Be honest! If a study was undertaken for a degree, it is normal for the supervisors to be named as second and third authors if they have had some input into at least editing the article. If they have not contributed anything to the article, they should be given acknowledgement but not authorship.

When there are a number of co-authors, the order of the names is considered important. As it is the lead clinical action researcher's project, they should be the first author because of their leading role in all aspects of study design, data collection and analysis, and article preparation. Co-authors should be listed in the order in which they have contributed. If, however, a lead action researcher delegates most of the article preparation to someone else in the project, then that person could legitimately take first authorship, as showing authorship is concerned with establishing responsibility for the resulting published paper rather than the project. In academic life, as can also be the case for practitioners, being seen to lead project teams and publish as first or second author are important in career terms. There may be heated debates about who takes precedence and why, so these aspects should be discussed and agreed by the team of co-authors before the paper is submitted.

Conflict of interest. This is more usually about stating publicly whether any authors have been, for example, funded by a drugs company to carry out the research, but in clinical action research studies it might be relevant to say that the lead researcher was, for example, Assistant Director of Nursing in the Trust. This should also be stated in the local context discussion in the introduction.

Copyright. You will be asked to sign copyright to the publishing journal, meaning that you assign rights to the journal to control and distribute the work. You should do this (or your work will not be published). You still maintain some rights over the use of the article, depending on the publisher's agreement, and will still be named as an original author. This copyright assignment protects the journal from you submitting the same piece elsewhere, as this would be an infringement of the agreement. It also gives the journal exclusive rights to disseminate your work widely, including internationally (Webb 2009).

Lastly, publication in journals may seem daunting! However, if you have carried out a project, whether you have been externally funded, or completed it as part of a qualification, or as part of a work role, you have a professional responsibility to write about it and make it available widely. You need to protect the anonymity of participants as consequences may follow from their identification (Williamson and Prosser 2002), although participants may waive these rights (see Chapter 7). Your work may be of interest and relevance to someone else in the field and you should disseminate it as widely as you can (see also Chapter 9). Clinical action research is about significant change and development for patient benefit, and generating new knowledge, and if you have been involved in these activities the world needs to know! It is equally important for the world of healthcare to publish studies which provide knowledge regarding why clinical change and development did not happen.

Summary

This chapter has examined how to write up action research projects in different ways for different audiences, including the requirements for writing an internal report, a dissertation or thesis, and a journal article. Reading all three sections provides insight and understanding of the challenges, criticism and creativity that surrounds the writing of clinical action research projects. The process, outcomes and key messages of the project need to be conveyed in appropriate ways to meet the needs of the readership. Readers will be senior health service managers, clinical colleagues, service users and carers, students, doctoral examiners and academic colleagues, and are a diverse readership. You need to write for that readership.

Practice, patience and perseverance is required as you undertake the writing process. As you draft and redraft your article, internal or academic report, never give up and remember:

> Nothing you write, if you hope to be good, will ever come out as you first hoped. (Lillian Hellman undated)

Useful websites and resources

FoNS (Foundation of Nursing Studies) *Centre for Nursing Innovation*: www.fons.org/

The aims of FoNS are to inspire and enable nurses to lead innovation and change in nursing and healthcare practice to improve patient care. Within the Centre for Nursing Innovation you can contribute to the International Practice Development Journal and access their action research short reports.

Steinberg Collection of nursing research: www.rcn.org.uk/development/library_steinberg_collection_of_nursing_research.

The RCN Steinberg Collection is a unique reference collection of over 1,000 UK doctoral theses from the 1950s to the present day completed by nurses and others on topics of relevance to nursing. It now contains a number of action research studies.

Webb, C (2009) *Writing for publication*. Oxford: Wiley-Blackwell. This booklet is available via the *Nurse Author and Editor* journal website at http://www.nurseauthoreditor.com. You will need to register with the website but this is free.

References

Bellman, L (2003) *Nurse-led change and development in clinical pactice*. Nursing Research Series. London: Wiley-Blackwell.

Bellman, L and Corrigan, P (2010) Using action research to develop a thoracic support nurse role to enhance quality of care. *Nursing Times* 106 (22) (8–14 June): 18–21.

Bellman, L and Wiseman, T (2010) Exploring nurse/midwifery leadership in using and doing research in clinical practice: Phase 1. University College London Hospitals NHS Foundation Trust, unpublished report.

Carter, P (2007) The importance of research in nursing. *Journal of Research in Nursing* 12(3): 207–208.

Darzi, Lord (2008) *High quality care for all: NHS next stage review. Final report*. London: Department of Health/The Stationery Office.

Department of Health (2010) *Equity and excellence: Liberating the NHS*. White paper. London: Department of Health/The Stationery Office.

Gray, D E (2009) *Doing research in the real world* (2nd edition). London: Sage.

Higgs, J and Titchen A (2001) *Professional practice in health, education and the creative arts*. Oxford: Blackwell Science.

Jackson, C and Butterworth, T (2007) Everyone's business, no-one's responsibility: Reporting clinical academic research activity by nurses in the United Kingdom. *Journal of Research in Nursing* 12(3): 213–223.

Lee, A (1998) Doctoral research as writing. In J Higgs and A Titchen (eds), *Practical knowledge and expertise in the health professions*. Oxford: Butterworth-Heinemann.

McCance, T, Fitzsimons, D and Armstrong, N C (2006) Developing a best practice framework to benchmark research and development activity in nursing and midwifery. *Journal of Research in Nursing* 11(2): 160–171.

McNiff, J and Whitehead, J (2009) *Doing and writing action research*. London: Sage.

Stringer, E (2007) *Action research* (3rd edition). London: Sage.

UniSA (2010) http://www.unisa.edu.au/resdegrees/candidates/thesis.asp (last accessed 1/11/2010).

Webb, C (2009) *Writing for publication*. Oxford: Wiley-Blackwell.

Webster, J (2007) Person-centred assessment with older people: An action research study to explore registered nurses of person-centred assessment within a framework of emancipatory practice development. Unpublished PhD thesis, University of Portsmouth, Portsmouth, UK.

Williamson, G R (2004): Developing lecturer practitioner roles in nursing using action research. Unpublished PhD thesis, University of Plymouth, Plymouth.

Williamson, G R and Prosser, S (2002) Action research: Politics, ethics and participation. *Journal of Advanced Nursing* 40(5): 587–593.

Winter, R and Munn-Giddings, C (2001) *A handbook for action research in health and social care*. London: Routledge.

9

PRESENTING CLINICAL ACTION RESEARCH STUDIES TO MIXED AUDIENCES

Loretta Bellman

Presenting your action research study to a range of audiences is an important part of the research process. Chapter 8 considered the writing of action research studies. You also have a responsibility to share new knowledge by direct engagement with professional colleagues as well as non-technical audiences. Oral presentation to mixed audiences is an important process which includes the opportunity for discussion and responding to questions, as well as receiving constructive criticism. If you are studying for a higher degree, it can also support preparation for the academic review process and the final *viva voce*. Unless in an examination setting, what you choose to present will depend on the study and the messages you wish to impart to your audience. However, it is important to recognise that there are still many people who have no knowledge of the methodology, so your presentation will also contribute to your audiences' exposure to action research:

> Why is it that I received no exposure to action research whatsoever before my doctoral studies? (Bradbury Huang 2010: 210)

Open access to new media content and discussion spaces, such as blogs, wikis, discussion boards and community networks, is becoming an important platform for many forms of inquiry in democratic societies (Hearn et al. 2009). Also, there are free online learning tools, such as the Effective Technical Presentations module (ASME Professional Practice Curriculum, available online, 2010 a–e), which underpins the content for this chapter. The use of these media sources provides further opportunities within which to publicise and present your project. You should also consider the mass (or old) media. How ready are you to share key aspects of your study with radio and television audiences? Apart from professional and stakeholder written accounts (Chapter 8), you may also like to consider newspaper and popular magazine audiences. Whatever medium you may choose, presentations need to be made interesting and engaging for diverse audiences.

Chapter objectives

This chapter will explore how to make your study appeal to mixed audiences through:

- knowing your audience;
- knowing the qualities of effective presentation;
- understanding new media and the mass media.

Knowing your audience

There are many different types of audience. Some groups may be eager to embrace your words, while others may be highly resistant. Just as in writing for different audiences, so you should ensure that your presentation will meet the needs of your audience. Indeed, if you have not considered your audience, you can plan what you believe to be an excellent presentation but you may discover a disinterested audience with little or no response to your efforts. For example, Buchanan et al. (2007) state that it should be evident that researchers and their practitioner audiences must appreciate each other's methodologies. Yet, the authors also acknowledge that healthcare researchers using qualitative perspectives will have problems communicating with healthcare practitioners with experience only of double-blind, randomised control trial methodology. The action researcher may of course have problems communicating with both – with the scientific community and even with some social scientists. Bradbury Huang (2010) cautions that with 'very conventional' social scientists it is important to educate them about the participative dimension of action research. So how do you know what your audience wants to know and what they are interested in? Audience types range from favourable to hostile and within any one audience there will often be a mixture of types (Box 9.1).

Box 9.1

Different types of audience (adapted from ASME Professional Practice Curriculum (2010a) 'Know Your Audience', © ASME.

Audience type	Position
Favourable	Already has some knowledge of the subject and are informed of your objectives for speaking. They are supportive of you, wish to learn about your specific topic and more about using the methodology.
Uninformed	Not familiar with your work. They may have a preconceived attitude toward your subject and feelings which might include apprehension, confusion or impatience.
Apathetic	Indifferent to your subject matter and do not wish to be involved in it. They may also be unknowledgeable about your subject matter.
Hostile	Hostile to your subject matter and/or the position you take.

A favourable audience will be supportive of your project. If this audience's prior knowledge makes you feel apprehensive, then in your introduction briefly state the extent of your action research experience while acknowledging their expertise. Remember that only you and your co-researchers know the full extent of your project so a favourable audience will also be focused on, and supportive of, your subject matter.

••• REFLECTIVE ACTIVITY 9.1 •••

Reflect on Box 9.1 and consider how you could overcome indifference and resistance within uninformed, apathetic and hostile members of an audience. Also consider what general information within action research methodology needs to be conveyed to mixed audiences.

Try to explore beforehand what uninformed, apathetic and even hostile members of an audience value, their beliefs and needs. A challenge is to try to connect them to your topic. Also, there will be preconceived ideas of your subject matter and the methodology. Experienced healthcare professionals sometimes believe that they know or can second guess the opinions of professional colleagues, other healthcare professionals and patient/carer views so beware of making assumptions. Whenever possible check out perceptions through, for example: direct contact, professional journals, websites, popular magazines. Find out as much as possible about your audience from whoever has asked you to make the presentation. Also, discuss the objectives of your presentation. The title of your talk is equally important; try to make it both interesting and intriguing. The title: 'Courage, faith and chocolate cake: professionalism in action' (Bellman 2001) described a politically challenging action research study which was presented to a mixed audience of healthcare professionals and non-healthcare academic staff at a research conference.

You will need to educate or re-educate uninformed and apathetic audience members. Consider using aspects of educational theory (Kaufman et al. 2000): in the introduction, try to engage the audience by relating your project to things they already know. Provide clear explanations to enable your audience to build new knowledge on to their current understanding and experiences. If sufficient time is available, ask members to reflect on their practice and past experiences and encourage personal contributions. For hostile members of an audience, try to explore, preferably in advance, any points of agreement. Be open to using the presentation as a springboard for understanding why they are hostile (if not known), and how your position might also shift to better incorporate their perspective. Try not to be defensive when there are, for example, dismissive remarks regarding action research not being real research compared to positivist approaches. Be prepared to argue your corner, including gaining their agreement that it is the research question/objectives that direct the researcher to adopt the most appropriate research methodology.

Whichever type of audience you present to, it is important to reinforce the following three main points:

- action research is a research methodology to systematically explore change and development in practice settings;
- the focus is on patient-centred outcomes and quality improvement;
- frontline staff are enabled to effect change with and for patients through the integration of collaboration, facilitation and empowerment.

According to Bradbury Huang (2010), the action researcher must develop a facility in communicating with two audiences: the local practitioners and the cosmopolitan community of scholars. Local practitioners are healthcare professionals. These professionals plus managers, patients, carers and academic partners all make up the local community. Generally speaking, communicating with the local community first provides an opportunity for validating and disseminating local learning (Bradbury Huang 2010). Yet, whether presenting to the local community or a community of scholars, you will need to know your audience and anticipate responding to both supportive and unfavourable reactions to your project.

How you introduce action research methodology will depend very much on your audience. Similar to writing up an account of action research, an effective presentation also requires much consideration and creativity. Action research is a complex process. It is not amenable to critique by the strategies used for other methodologies; the term is rarely used in the management and organisational change literature, and where it is discussed, it is presented in very different language (Badger 2000). For managers, the term 'organisational change' will be very familiar but may receive a mixed reaction. The 'Look–Think–Act' routine (Box 9.2) described by Stringer (2007) can be a user-friendly way of presenting the methodology. Kemmis and McTaggart (1999) refer to the Plan, Act, Observe, Reflect spiral of activity. However you describe action research, it is most definitely not a neat, orderly activity that enables participants to proceed in a step-by-step manner. People often work backwards, may have to repeat processes, revise procedures, rethink interpretations, leapfrog steps or stages, and sometimes make radical changes in direction (Stringer 2007: 9).

Box 9.2

Look-Think-Act – a basic action research routine (Stringer 2007)

Look	Gather relevant information (Gather data) Build a picture: describe the situation (Define and describe)
Think	Explore and analyse: What is happening here? (Analyse) Interpret and explain: How/why are things as they are? (Theorise)
Act	Plan Implement Evaluate

The qualities of effective presentation

We have all been to presentations which we have considered very informative, motivating, even inspirational. Likewise, we have all witnessed presentations that have left us feeling frustrated, patronised and none the wiser.

• • • REFLECTIVE ACTIVITY 9.2 • • •

Recall a presentation that you enjoyed and which increased your understanding and motivated you in some way. Jot down what you consider to be the qualities of an effective presentation.

An effective presentation is one which is well paced, clearly spoken and flows smoothly from one aspect to another, where visual aids are used appropriately, and which captures the attention of the audience throughout. Style, pacing and flow are key qualities of an effective presentation. There are five elements of style (Box 9.3). A flat, monotone delivery will quickly lose your audience. If you speak too quickly your audience may not be able to process all the information you present. Speaking fast can also be an overt sign of nervousness. Almost every public speaker, no matter how experienced, feels some degree of nervousness. One way of dealing with the situation is to acknowledge that having some nerves is important to improving performance (Gray 2009).

Box 9.3

The elements of style (adapted from ASME Professional Practice Curriculum (2010b), 'Qualities of an Effective Speech', © ASME

Element of Style	Description
Colour of language	Indicates descriptiveness: your choice of adjectives, adverbs, verbs and nouns, showing the extent to which your words are evocative and explicit.
Vocal dynamics	Describes how you use your voice: intonation (pitch), loudness, and the speed of your speech. Use your voice like an instrument to project sound, change tone and increase tempo.
Accent	Your accent is a key feature that distinguishes you from others. It can be a positive quality or an impediment to communication. Using visual aids will help the audience to 'hear' your ideas better.
Body language	There are many non-verbal aspects in a presentation: posture, facial expression, eye contact, the way you use your hands, and the extent to which you move around during the presentation.
Attitude	Attitude is an integral part of style. Negative behaviours include arrogance, indifference, insincerity, abrasiveness and over-aggressiveness. Positive behaviours include enthusiasm, passion, humour, empathy and sincerity.

The basic structure of a good presentation is to have an introduction, a middle and an end. The introduction enables you to 'connect' with your audience (Gray 2009). You (and co-presenters if present) may wish to briefly establish your identity and credibility to discuss the project. You should try to ensure that in the middle part of the presentation each point flows effortlessly into the next. The themes of the action research process should enable a logical flow, for example: initiating the study; engaging with co-researchers; identifying the topic; seeking ethical approval; identifying research methods, etc. Ways to enhance the flow are through enlarging, magnifying, refuting, relating and reinforcing your point (Box 9.4).

Box 9.4

Ways to enhance the flow of a presentation (adapted from ASME Professional Practice Curriculum (2010b), 'Qualities of an Effective Speech', © ASME

Enhancing Flow	Examples
Enlarge your point	This can simplify ideas and make it easier to understand: • In the broader perspective • On a larger level • In the broader sense • In the grand scheme of things • We have seen this on a larger scale.
Magnify your point	This brings your information into further focus: For example • At a closer glance • On a smaller level • Let's take a closer look
Refute your point	When presenting a perspective that is opposite to what you have just said: • On the other hand • In an opposite sense • Conversely • The disadvantages are • The advantages are
Relate and reinforce your point	This also helps you to make your point in another way: • On another level • In another way • Similarly • In the same sense • How many of you have ever experienced

The factor that sinks more presentations than any other is the sheer volume of information bad presenters try to convey (Gray 2009). As listeners are only capable of remembering two or three key messages, make sure these are crystal clear. You can reinforce your key messages to more people more effectively by using a 'hook' and analogy. A hook is a powerful statement, word or phrase that stands out like a headline. The hook should be very brief, something that is easy to remember and that connects with different parts of the presentation. It could even be part of the title of a presentation, as in the above example: 'Courage, faith and chocolate cake'. You reinforce the hook through each stage of the action research process as appropriate.

Analogy is a useful device to employ to reinforce your point. It enables your audience to appreciate the point you are making and it creates a strong visual image. Action research examples could be: getting some clinical colleagues to change their mind was like pulling teeth; while appearing enthusiastic to participate, trying to get this group of co-researchers together was like herding cats; inviting patients to participate was essential but was like opening up a can of worms.

The end of the presentation requires you to not only summarise your two or three key points, but also to leave a strong impression with the audience. This stage of the presentation should be delivered with enthusiasm and energy (Gray 2009). Think of your conclusion as a small package of ideas that you wish the audience to take away with them. You may also choose to do one of following:

- Turn the subject back on the audience. Leave them with a question to consider. For example: imagine that your presentation supported the assertion by Milner et al. (2005: 911) that the limited research assessing nurse educators' influence on the professional development of practising nurses, including the use of research findings, is alarming. The question to leave the audience with may be: How can nurse educators adopt a clinical academic approach to using and doing research with nurses in clinical practice settings?
- End with a quotation that distils your idea eloquently, possibly on a broader, more universal level. For example:
    - Anton Chekov's 'Knowledge is of no value unless you put it into practice' (Anton Chekov Infosite 2010);
    - Kurt Levin's 'If you want to truly understand something try to change it' (Skills2Lead 2010);
    - Charles Darwin's 'It is not the strongest of the species that survives, nor the most intelligent that survives. It is the one that is the most adaptable to change' (Darwin 2010).
- Leave your audience with a responsibility and briefly indicate what that responsibility is and what they must do. For example: within the presentation

of two clinical action research projects (Bellman 2003) a key expressionvoiced by health service managers was that of 'eye-opener' regarding their surprise at the creative ability of their staff. Managers were initially somewhat reticent in relinquishing control to enable their staff to take the initiative in deciding the focus of the projects, but by doing so they were delighted with the improvements in patient care that resulted. Recommendations to the audience could therefore include managers adopting a transformational leadership approach by creating an environment in which their staff feel and are empowered to lead change and innovation in their practice settings.

- Leave your audience with an exciting thought, a vision of tomorrow, an assurance of achievement, or an affirmation that the right course of action was taken. For example: 'An unexpected outcome of our action research was the interest from staff in other clinical areas within the hospital. The innovation is now more widespread than we'd anticipated. ... Our future research endeavours will be well informed by the learning we have experienced in undertaking this study' (Smith et al. 2009: 19).

The effectiveness of your presentation can be gauged by the reaction of your audience. Four positive reactions may be experienced from an action research presentation: intellectual; emotional; memory; practical. Some examples can be found in Box 9.5. To be told that your presentation is inspirational can be the ultimate accolade.

Box 9.5

Anticipated positive audience reactions which may be reported during or following an action research presentation (ASME Professional Practice Curriculum (2010c), 'Communications Devices', © ASME

Listener's reaction	Examples
Intellectual	• I can relate to this issue. • I get it! This is just like that (from hearing an analogy). • Now I can visualise how this works. • By taking part in your hands-on example I understand how this works.
Emotional	• That's a really funny way of putting it. • I understand. This is very sad. • This information makes me excited for the future. • I am in awe of what people can create! • I want to be part of this cause.

(Continued)

(Continued)

Memory	• That's the third time you said it, I think I get it! • Now that you put it that way, I will remember this! • P.O.W.E.R – that's an easy acronym to remember. • That's a very memorable analogy. • When you put it that way, it's unforgettable!
Practical	• I can see how this can really be put to use in my work area. • I can use this for my own project. • This is much quicker and worthwhile. • I believe my colleagues and I can do this.

• • • REFLECTIVE ACTIVITY 9.3 • • •

In the preparation and review of your presentation, think of some analogies to describe aspects of your study. In what other ways can you deliver your key messages?

The message is not only limited to what you say but how you say it, so your 'tone' is equally important. Positive tone is energetic, friendly, humorous and clear as well as the way in which you project yourself in terms of emotion, attitude and personality. It is useful to consider counterproductive elements of tone. No doubt you have been confronted with some or all of the following negative elements of a person's tone (and not just during a presentation): condescension; egocentricity; abrasiveness or arrogance; exaggerated sincerity; authoritarian (Box 9.6). It is unnecessary, inappropriate and indeed doubtful that you will demonstrate any of these negative tones. The tones described are the antithesis to those needed to lead and facilitate a clinicalaction research study.

Box 9.6

Negative elements of a person's tone (ASME Professional Practice Curriculum (2010d), 'Other Communications Devices', © ASME

Negative elements	Impact
Condescension	When you assume a tone of condescension your audience will feel as if you are talking down to them. No matter how much mastery you have in your field, you should avoid taking a tone of superiority over your audience.

Egocentricity	Egocentricity is self-centeredness. If you use the words I, me, mine, my, or ours, we, us (if speaking of yourself or your organisation) too often your audience may feel too removed or excluded from your project.
Abrasiveness or arrogance	Arrogance, inflexibility and indifference to the ideas of others constitute some elements of an abrasive tone. Abrasive speakers also tend to be critical of other individuals and organisations. There is no reason for any presenter, no matter how highly esteemed in his/her field, to show a tone of arrogance. Your audience may not only resent you for this, but may even grow increasingly hostile during the presentation.
Exaggerated sincerity	It's one thing to express yourself in ways that are polite, pleasant and respectful to others. However, you will be viewed as fake and insincere if you overdo this tone.
Authoritarian	Some speakers have the problem of being too authoritarian in tone. They may state their opinions as facts and emphasise their approach as the *only* approach.

The use of visual aids

Visual aids have the capacity to enhance and enrich a presentation, but when not used well they have the capacity to wreck it (Gray 2009). There are many sources of visual aids, including trusty PowerPoint slides. However, how often have you watched a PowerPoint presentation and found that you could not read what was written on the slide; you could not clearly distinguish the colours of a pie chart; there was too much detail to decipher; you felt overwhelmed by the number of slides, etc.? Always aim for simplicity.

••• REFLECTIVE ACTIVITY 9.4 •••

You may know some of the deadly sins when using PowerPoint. Jot down as many as you can and then refer to Box 9.7

As well as the deadly sins, faulty audio-visual equipment can jeopardise a presentation. If possible for you and any co-presenters, it is worthwhile to visit the presentation site beforehand to check the equipment and the acoustics. Arrive early and if possible run through the presentation, especially if using video clips or CDs. Visiting the presentation room well in advance and checking the equipment can also help to calm your nerves and help you feel more confident (Gray 2009).

Box 9.7

Some of the deadly sins when using PowerPoint (Gray 2009)

The sin	The consequence
Using fonts that are too small	Inability of audience to read the information
Using endless bullet point slides	Complete audience boredom
Making slides busy and packed with text	Inability of audience to process the information
Using too many colours or inappropriate colours	Audience confusion
Using too many animation effects	Audience distraction or irritation
Facing the screen when talking, not the audience	Lack of 'connection' with the audience; less interest in the presentation
Flat, monotone delivery	Audience falls asleep or 'switches off'

Alternative communication devices

There are many ways in which you can attract and retain attention, including the use of alternative communication devices. These devices can also enable you to pitch the presentation appropriately for your audience. According to Stringer (2007) and Denzin (1997), it may be possible to present the outcomes of an action research process through:

- drama;
- role play;
- simulation;
- dance;
- song;
- poetry;
- works of art;
- a combination of the above.

These creative arts can be very effective complementary communication devices when engaging with different audiences. Titchen and Manley (2006) refer to the creative arts in their critical insight of their work as action researchers. The authors also acknowledge the increasing use of creative arts and artistic expression within aspects of the research process, including data gathering. Once again, knowing as much as possible about your audience will guide presentation decision making, as well as how comfortable you (and co-presenters) feel about using creative arts.

Introducing humour in a non-offensive way can be an appropriate device to animate a presentation, no matter how complex or abstract the point you are trying to make. Humour includes cartoons, amusing quotations, asides and jokes. These brief pauses in a presentation engage the audience and revive attentiveness. Humour is also a tool for relieving tension in situations where opposing points of view are present. While humour is a useful device it should not be overused. Care should be taken when choosing examples as what you consider amusing may backfire on you.

Effective presentation is a skill encompassing a novice to expert framework akin to the Dreyfus and Dreyfus model of skill acquisition (Dreyfus and Dreyfus 1986). As with learning any skill, the more you practise, the more skilled you become. Rehearse, with co-presenters, in front of colleagues who can provide you with constructive feedback. Positive thoughts will also enhance your presentation ability (Gray 2009):

- I have practised this. I am fluent.
- I am the expert in the room (regarding this study).
- I will command their attention.
- I know most of the answers. I can always open issues up for discussion.

New media and the mass media

New and the mass (or old) media can both play a significant part in enabling you to present your project to mixed audiences. New media sources, such as blogs, wikis, discussion boards, archive sharing areas and community networks, can provide many benefits for clinical action research projects, including improving networking, research collaboration and creative content development (Hearn et al. 2009). These new media sources also offer vast potential for presenting aspects of your research and the outcomes of your project, plus receiving feedback in less formal ways. A discussion forum, for example, allows for broadcast-style one-to-many and many-to-many modes of communication (Hearn et al. 2009). A discussion forum can be incorporated into a bespoke website for your project. A website is an innovative way to share a password-protected workspace with the co-researchers throughout the project, if all agree. Also, you can embrace a global audience by posting non-confidential aspects of the work in progress, as well as the final report, on another part of the same website.

• • • REFLECTIVE ACTIVITY 9.5 • • •

Explore the types of new media sources you could incorporate into your project. What are the pros and cons of using the new media sources you have identified?

The need to raise the profile of your project through the mass (or old) media of radio, television, newspapers and magazines should also be considered. Keep abreast of political and healthcare news. Information regarding your project will have a greater chance of acceptance if you can clearly demonstrate how it is newsworthy. Ways of accessing the mass media may include:

- personal initial contact via email or telephone. Provide a brief overview of the study in a user-friendly way, clearly pointing out your two or three key messages;
- via your professional or work organisation publicising your work and seeking access to the mass media on your behalf;
- if appropriate, by informing patient groups/charities of your project. Many charities have well-publicised annual collection weeks, information days and publicity events, e.g. from Parliamentary receptions and conferences to fun runs. Try to present your project information in time to coincide with a special event. The press officer of the charity can then advise you on how to proceed;
- sometimes reporters may already know of your work through accessing a website, your journal articles, from attending a formal presentation, etc., and will approach you.

Unlike professional discussions and formal presentations, mass media people control when and how your project is depicted. Also, air time is limited for radio and television and what you say is often edited. You must therefore be your own editor, ensuring that you provide the most precise, selective information, with little room for error or misinterpretation. As with all presentations, preparation is the key to success.

Preparing for radio and television interviews

From your repertoire as an experienced healthcare professional you will have many transferable communication skills to aid you in preparing for a media interview. In addition, you know the project thoroughly. Adopt a friendly, confident tone. If you appear ambiguous or ambivalent, you will not be an effective communicator. Let people know where you stand and why. Preparation for a media interview includes:

- determining who is the audience;
- preparing three main points;
- anticipating difficult questions;
- preparing 'people' stories;
- dressing appropriately.

In determining who the audience is, request the press or media kit of the organisation that plans to interview you. The demographic information on their audience may be useful for you. Also, find out who will interview you and, if possible, watch a programme they are presenting. As stated before, having three main points reflects the fact that people are only capable of remembering up to three key messages, so ensure these are crystal clear. To anticipate difficult questions, request a list of them in advance. Also, ask what type of information you will be expected to provide. Find out, if possible, who else is being interviewed or will be present and whether they support or refute action research. Write typical responses that you can memorise in advance. Try to include 'people' stories to elaborate your points in a more user-friendly way. It goes without saying that your dress should reflect the occasion and can also enhance your confidence.

Media people are always looking for a sound bite. A sound bite is the one line that crystallises what you wish to say; the statement that is packaged with clarity, succinctness and symbolism. It has impact, stands on its own and is easy to recall. Sound bites from a clinical action research study could include parts of the title or key themes that emerge from the analysed data. For example, any of the five key themes from an action research study (Bellman and Corrigan 2010) can be useful sound bites:

- it's the need to improve the quality of care;
- brought research to life;
- a rollercoaster of emotions and experiences;
- process is as important as outcome;
- we did it ourselves and learnt so much.

Ways of conveying a sound bite include leaving several seconds on either side of your statement to have impact. In a recorded interview, saying a sound bite slowly, and with emphasis, should ensure that the editor does not extract it from the tape. You may like to incorporate some poetics, a rhythmic quality to your statement. Try to make words colourful and meaningful, for example: *throughout the study we overdosed on 'courage, faith and chocolate cake'*. Also, using words and phrases such as *consequently, as a result of, on the one hand... on the other hand,* are transitional statements which can link one idea seamlessly to the next. By using transitions, you make it easier for people to follow your ideas. It will also be easier for editors to extract key statements in the right context. Another way of conveying a winning sound bite is to turn a statement into a provocative question. For example, you could say: *Recognition and support for practitioner-led research in clinical setting sis one of the most challenging issues in healthcare organisations today.* Or you could say: *The question for health service managers is do you want a disempowered workforce that has no incentive to explore change and innovation together for patient benefit?*

• • • REFLECTIVE ACTIVITY 9.6 • • •

Prepare some sound bites from your project by identifying certain statements that could be irresistible to the editors of media sources.

Summary

Preparation and rehearsal time are required to deliver an effective action research project presentation to mixed audiences. You should explore, whenever possible, the needs of your audience and use appropriate jargon-free language in creative ways. The audience often includes people who have little or no knowledge of clinical action research. Demonstrating the democratic, participatory, liberating and life-enhancing approach to research (Stringer 2007) may be possible. However, even if these key tenets are less evident in your study, you still need to embrace the methodology and present it in a meaningful and non-patronising way for your audience. New media and the mass media forms of communication should also be embraced as contemporary ways of presenting to much wider audiences as well as receiving feedback and recognition of your work. Clinical action researchers have a responsibility to disseminate their work to a wide audience. You never know just how positive and influential the impact of your presentation can be until you try it.

Useful websites and resources

ASME Professional Practice Curriculum available online (2010): http://professional-practice.asme.org/Communications/NonTech/Introduction.cfm

Foundation of Nursing Studies (FoNS): www.fons.org/

FoNS has a virtual space for you to explore, exchange, share, collaborate and develop. Their Common Room enables you to make contact with other people who are undertaking similar work to yourself.

Royal College of Nursing: www.rcn.org/uk/

Many aspects of presentations can be found by searching the Royal College of Nursing website. For example: Top Tips for Speaking at Congress; in the Political Leadership programme; and the Welsh Board's free one-day intensive media training for nurses interested in speaking to the media.

References

Anton Chekov Infosite (2010) www.antonchekov.net/more.htm/ (accessed 17/07/2010).

ASME Professional Practice Curriculum (2010a) *Communicating to non-technical audiences*. © ASME. Available at: http://professionalpractice.asme.org/Communications/NonTech/Introduction.cfm (accessed 1/7/2010).

ASME Professional Practice Curriculum) (2010b) *Know your audience*. © ASME.Available at: http://professionalpractice.asme.org/Communications/NonTech/Know_Audience.cfm (accessed 1/7/2010).

ASME Professional Practice Curriculum) (2010c) *Qualities of an effective speech*. © ASME. Available at: http://professionalpractice.asme.org/Communications/NonTech/Qualities_Effective_Speech.cfm (accessed 1/7/2010).

ASME Professional Practice Curriculum) (2010d) *Communications devices*. © ASME. Available at: http://professionalpractice.asme.org/Communications/NonTech/Communications_Devices.cfm (accessed 1/7/2010).

ASME Professional Practice Curriculum) (2010e) *Other communications devices*. © ASME. Available at: http://professionalpractice.asme.org/Communications/NonTech/Communications Devices 2.cfm (accessed 1/7/2010).

Badger, T G (2000) Action research, change and methodological rigour. *Journal of Nursing Management* 8: 201–207.

Bellman, L (2001) Courage, faith and chocolate cake: Requisites for exploring professionalism in action. *Educational Action Research* 9(2): 225–242. DOI: 10.1080/09650790100200147.

Bellman, L (2003) *Nurse-led change and development in clinical practice*. Nursing Research Series. London: Wiley-Blackwell.

Bellman, L and Corrigan, P (2010) Using action research to develop a thoracic support nurse role to enhance quality of care. *Nursing Times* (8–14 June) 106(22): 18–21.

Bradbury Huang, H (2010) What is good action research? Why the resurgent interest? *Action Research* 8: 93. DOI: 10.1177/1476750310362435.

Buchanan, DA, Fitzgerald, L and Ketley, D (eds) (2007) *The sustainability and spread of organisational change*. London: Routledge.

Darwin, C (2010) Charles Darwin, http://en.wikiquote.org/wiki/Charles_Darwin (accessed 17/07/2010).

Denzin, NK (1997) *Interpretive ethnography*. Thousand Oaks, CA: Sage.

Dreyfus, H L and Dreyfus, S E (1986) *Mind over machine: The power of human intuition and expertise in the age of the computer*. Oxford: BasilBlackwell.

Gray, D E (2009) *Doing research in the real world* (2nd edition). London: Sage.

Hearn, G, Tacchi, J, Foth, M and Lennie, J (2009) *Action research and new media*. Cresskill, NJ: Hampton Press.

Kaufman, D M, Mann, K V and Jennett, P A (2000) *Teaching and learning in medical education: How theory can inform practice*. Medical Education Occasional Publication. Edinburgh: Association for the Study of Medical Education.

Kemmis, S and McTaggert, R (1999) *The action research planner* (3rd edition). Geelong, Vic.: Deakin University Press.

Milner, F M, Estabrooks, C and Humphrey, C (2005) Clinical nurse educators as agents for change: Increasing research utilisation. *International Journal of Nursing Studies* 42(8): 899–914.

Skills2Lead (2010) www.Skills2Lead.com/quotes-about-change.html (accessed 17/07/2010).

Smith, S, Lewis, P and Wilson, V (2009) A 'wee' problem: Using action research to facilitate a change in urine collection methods. *Neonatal, Paediatric and Child Health Nursing* 12(1): 15–19.

Stringer, E (2007) *Action research* (3rd edition). London: Sage.

Titchen, A and Manley, K (2006) Spiralling towards transformational action research: Philosophical and practical journeys. *Educational Action Research* 14(3): 333–356.

10

EVALUATING THE QUALITY OF ACTION RESEARCH PROJECTS

Graham R Williamson

Action researchers, funding bodies, ethics committees, participants and readers need a shared understanding of how to evaluate the quality of action research proposals, projects and written reports. This is not as straightforward as it might sound as some argue (Bradbury and Reason 2006; Koch and Kralik 2006) that the quality of action research is very contextually-based, and that is it problematic to try to ascribe quality criteria to such activity.

Chapter objectives

This chapter will briefly:

- examine ideas concerning quality criteria, drawing together some authors' views about what constitutes 'good' or 'high quality' action research;
- outline their ideas in the form of 'tools' that can be used for critical reading and reviewing projects and proposals;
- invite you to review three studies from different locations around the world using the critiquing frameworks outlined. Short commentaries are provided on these studies, based on the evaluative ideas outlined in the chapter.

Introduction: why have criteria to evaluate action research?

Elliott (2007; following Stake and Schwandt 2006) argues that there are two opposing views of quality: quality-as-experienced (resulting from immediate experience) and quality-as-measured (in relation to externally agreed criteria or constructs). The role of the person evaluating an activity is thus different in each view, so that quality can be experienced as a direct result of personal experience or measured against a list, or possibly both. To evaluate the quality of something from personal experience is highly subjective and may require in-depth analysis, whereas evaluating something based on objective criteria requires greater detachment and can involve reducing it to an overall 'score'. Participants in action research studies will have a different experience of the quality of their project than detached readers of the project reports. Few people are directly involved in action research compared to the numbers of potential readers, particularly when a project is written up as a journal article (see also Chapter 8), but even so there is distrust of 'checklists' or 'rules' for evaluating quality among action researchers (Bradbury and Reason 2006; Koch and Kralik 2006).

••• REFLECTIVE ACTIVITY 10.1 •••

Consider the following questions:

1 Why is it necessary to evaluate action research studies?
2 Whose needs would evaluating action research serve?
3 Why might some people disagree with evaluative criteria for AR?

••• SUGGESTIONS TO ANSWER REFLECTIVE ACTIVITY 10.1 •••

1 Why is it necessary to evaluate action research studies?
With the current movement in healthcare research for evidence-based practice, research papers are receiving much scrutiny for their quality and application to practice, and arguably action research must also be open to evaluation if it is to be considered as evidence for practice, which primarily must be to change practice for patient benefit.

2 Whose needs would evaluating action research serve?
The provision of quality criteria for action research can serve the needs of funders as much research is carried out as a result of researchers securing research funding from external sources. Funders will want to know how to decide which studies to pay for and whether the end products were beneficial to readers. As those reading action research studies may know little about action research as a methodology, they may benefit from a set of evaluative criteria.

- Practitioners
  - as those seeking to change practice may be considering whether action research studies could be applied to their own areas (have transferability) and may welcome evaluative criteria.

- Authors and editors
  - as most journals carry sections on how to write papers and reports, but not many carry specific instructions for action researchers. The Sage journal *Action Research* is one exception (available from the journal website at http://arj.sagepub.com/). Their criteria are as follows:
    - Articulation of objectives
    - Evidence of partnership and participation
    - Contribution to action research theory/practice
    - Clear and explicit methods and process
    - Actionability (useful new ideas)
    - **Reflexivity**
    - Significance (the ideas have a meaning beyond their context)
- It would be helpful for authors and editors to have shared criteria for action research, as exists for reporting randomised controlled trials (see CONSORT at: http://www.consort-statement.org/).
- Students and their supervisors
  - If students are undertaking action research for postgraduate study, their work will need to meet quality academic standards, including questions like 'How do we know your work is of an appropriate standard?' Addressing this question increases understanding for both the student and their supervisor, particularly if the supervisor has little or no experience of action research methodology.
- Critics
  - Those who are critical of action research as lacking 'rigour' (in their terms) could use the criteria to understand more fully the strengths of action research.

3 Why might some people disagree with evaluative criteria for AR?

Some people disagree with having evaluative criteria for AR as AR studies are highly contextual and specific to their local area. It could be argued that their quality can only be fully understood by those directly involved: that their quality is dependent on quality-as-experienced rather than quality-as-measured.

Even if action researchers are reluctant to use quantitative or rules-based approaches, many authors refer to some form of quality assessment in their work, whether this is discussed as 'validity', 'rigour', 'guidance for assessment' or some other evaluative term. This may seem surprising given the quantitative roots of the term 'validity'. The issue of **validity** has been discussed extensively in Chapter 2 and will not be revisited here. Instead the work of some key authors in relation to the broader issue of quality in action research will be examined.

• • • REFLECTIVE ACTIVITY 10.2 • • •

Reflect on AR work that you have read or been involved with and develop your own criteria for judging AR studies. Compare your criteria with the views of various authors below.

Tools to evaluate the quality of action research

Herr and Anderson (2005) note that trustworthiness and credibility are terms that have been used to evaluate action research (and see the discussion in Chapter 2), but choose to use '**validity**' as a more recognisable term, even if it does not have the same meaning for action researchers as in other types of research. Instead, they argue that there are five goals of action research, and they link these to five types of **validity** (Table 10.1).

Koch and Kralik (2006) discuss rigour and quality in action research, arguing that there are sufficient rules-based approaches to rigour but that what is important in action research is whether it is accessible, makes a difference and is sustainable. They note that during the 1980s writers struggled to apply quantitative criteria, including **validity**, to action research work, but that since then qualitative concepts, such as credibility, transferability and dependability, have been developed from the work of Guba and Lincoln (1989) and others.

Koch and Kralik (2006) pose the questions set out in Table 10.2 for consideration regarding the rigour of AR (Table 10.2).

Table 10.1 Goals of action research and their link to quality criteria (adapted from Herr and Anderson 2005: 55)

Goals of action research	Quality/validity criteria
1. Generation of new knowledge	Process validity: Has an appropriate sequence of events, such as reflective cycling, taken place? What other data are discussed? Dialogic validity: Has peer review taken place for academic theses and journal articles?
2. Achievement of action-oriented outcomes	Outcome validity: Have things changed? Have problems been reframed?
3. 'Education' of researcher and participants	Catalytic validity: How have their views on social reality altered?
4. Results are relevant to the local setting	Democratic validity: Has genuine participation taken place?
5. Sound and appropriate research methodology	Process validity: Is the research process sound?

Table 10.2 Koch and Kralik's questions regarding rigour (adapted from Koch and Kralik 2006)

Question	Explanation
1 What is the worldview?	An authentic desire to secure useful information that makes a difference to all stakeholders in healthcare, particularly clients and the community. It may not always be possible to effect beneficial change, but participation is a central requirement.
2 Is the inquiry credible?	People's voices must be represented adequately and so their stories must be allowed to emerge in meaningful narratives which make experiences come alive. Participants are part of the validation process, so credibility exists when the multiple voices of participants emerge that are grounded in the data.
3 Is the inquiry transferable?	Transferability is in evidence when readers have enough contextual information to be able to make a judgement about whether it can be relevant to their own setting. This is relevant not necessarily for the substance of the study but for the theoretical ideas generated.
4 Is the study dependable?	Can the process be audited? Using systematic processes for data collection and analysis means that decisions are clear and can be shown to be so.
5 Is the study believable?	Is there clear reflexivity? Have authors demonstrated that they have considered and discussed their relationship with the research and its impact on them and their thinking?
6 What values and interests do researchers bring to the inquiry?	Are any values and interests acknowledged and declared in publications? Everyone brings these to research and they should not be allowed to unduly influence things.
7 Is the work accessible?	Although a text should be co-constructed with participants, it is the researchers' responsibility to bring the work together. The work needs to be engaging so that people will read it.

Gomm et al. (2000) argue that, as a term, 'rigour' is now so widely applied as to be virtually meaningless. Even so, they produce a list of questions to be used for evaluating its quality (see Table 10.3a).

For Coghlan and Brannick (2010), rigour in AR depends on four processes. These are:

- multiple 'cycling' and accurate recording of this process;
- discussion of how the project has challenged and developed the thinking of the researcher and participants;
- how different views about events are accessed to produce confirming and disconfirming evidence; and
- how the project interpretations and diagnoses are supported and challenged, and how theoretical and philosophical frameworks underpin the ideas and the project.

Table 10.3a Gomm et al.'s questions for evaluating the quality of action research (adapted from Gomm et al. 2000)

Questions	Issues
1 **Evidence of change** Is there evidence that the action has taken place because of the 'intervention'? How has the situation before and after the study been described? Are effects for all those involved discussed?	What measures or criteria have been used to demonstrate the research claims? Is testimonial evidence reliable or is there a one-sided perspective which only shows the project in a good light?
2 **Replicability** Could a similar project be undertaken elsewhere? Including: • what was done? • characteristics of all those involved • resourcing • local context.	As action research involves complex change scenarios, is enough detail included for readers to judge the extent of transferability?
3 **'Experiment effect'** Is it clear how much the intervention and/ or how much the energy and enthusiasm of those involved contributed to the change?	Enthusiasm may be enough, but an effective change strategy would be needed for transferability.
4 **Biased reporting** How likely is it that the report was written to give the project a favourable light?	As collaborative projects, action research reports are likely to represent consensus between participants, and may not represent the full story.
5 **Insight and understanding** How much of each are proffered which may improve practice elsewhere?	Is there clear transferability?

An influential conception of quality issues in action research, which is also quoted elsewhere (e.g. Herr and Anderson 2005; Koch and Kralik 2006) is that of Bradbury and Reason (2006). They extend the debate by arguing that central to the quality of AR is the philosophical question: How do action researchers know that they are actually doing '*good work*'? They discuss five choice-points in a 'participatory worldview', which, they argue, broadens the 'bandwidth' about what is good quality research. The five choices are:

- that action researchers must examine the quality of their participation in relation to the work they accomplish: participants should be energised and empowered by being involved, and should gain new insight and understanding into their worlds and a critical consciousness;
- that action researchers should ask whether the work is useful and helpful: 'Do people whose reputations and livelihoods are at stake act differently as a result of the work?' This requires action researchers to ask

pragmatic questions about their work and be reflexive about the answers they receive;

- that action researchers should acknowledge that they need both conceptual knowledge and participation, but as the work progresses through the various cycles they also need to be clear that any new knowledge is appropriately grounded in the contextual experience;that inquiry methods should be appropriate to the work and researchers should use a variety of data collection methods drawn from different methodological traditions to gain the fullest perspective;that the wider context of the AR project is an important aspect of validity: 'To what extent does the project "change the world"?' As micro and macrolevels are intimately connected, AR should enable participants to live a better life in organisations and in a general sense;
- that participation needs to be continued into the future, not just for the length of the project, and a living interest needs to be created which survives the researcher's interest.

Bradbury and Reason's (2006) five choice-points overlap and are relevant to individual researchers in different measures: no AR project will be able to address them all, let alone equally, and each project articulates its own standards. However, researchers must make explicit which of the choice-points are important in their work, and demonstrate their achievement by discussing the strengths and weaknesses of the work in relation to the choice-points they identify. These are summarised in Table 10.4a.

Waterman et al. (2001) argue that although it may seem an anathema to the flexible and **democratic** traditions of action research, guidance on the assessment of action research quality is necessary for the sake of clarity, to encourage novice researchers to achieve high standards, and to encourage reporting standards in journals. They stop short of designing a checklist with a numerical scoring system, tailoring their guidance to researchers as well as funders and putting forward 20 questions. While some elements are common to all research, those which are particularly relevant for action research are marked with an asterisk (*) (see Table 10.5a).

Table 10.4 Issues as choice-points and questions for quality in action research (adapted from Bradbury and Reason 2006: 350)

- Explicit development of praxis and participation
- Guided by concern for outcomes
- Includes a variety of forms of investigation
- Worthy of the term 'significant'
- Developing new infrastructures for working practices

Table 10.5a 20 questions for judging the rigour of action research (adapted from Waterman et al. 2001)

Question	Explanation
1 *Are the aims and objectives of each stage of the research clearly stated?*	Did the authors of the project clearly define the aims and objectives of the project and were they appropriate?
2 *Was the action research relevant to practitioners and/or users?*	Action research should: address local issues; contribute to new understanding; be relevant to participants; suggest further research and make recommendations for policy and practice.
3 **Were the phases of the project clearly outlined?*	Was a logical process in evidence (or intended)? Should include: • problem identification • planning • action • evaluation.
4 **Were the participants and stakeholders clearly described and justified?*	Did the project focus on service users and/or health professionals? How were participants selected and recruited for each phase of the project?
5 **Was consideration given to the local context while implementing change?*	Contextual factors should be discussed, such as why it was selected, and a critical examination of values, beliefs and power relationships should be included.
6 **Was the relationship between researchers and participants adequately considered?*	The level and extent of participation should be clearly defined for each stage; there should be reflexivity by all involved?
7 *Was the project managed appropriately?*	Key persons in organisations should have been involved; those involved need requisite skills to implement change and/or research; implementation plans should be feasible, achievable, and clearly a result of local participation.
8 *Were ethical issues encountered and how were they dealt with?*	Rights of participants, researchers and those affected by the action research process all require consideration, including confidentiality and informed consent.
9 *Was the study adequately funded/supported?*	Were the assessments of cost and resources realistic? Were there any conflicts of interest?
10 *Was the length and timetable of the project realistic?*	Was the project completed on time? Was there slippage of the timeline?
11 *Were data collected in a way that addressed the research issue?*	Were appropriate research methodologies, methods of data collection and analysis used to answer research questions?
12 *Were steps taken to promote the rigour of the findings?*	Differing perspectives on issues should be used, as should method and theoretical triangulation. Key findings should be fed back to participants and their feedback used. Reflexive accounts should be offered.
13 *Were data analyses sufficiently rigorous?*	Were procedures for analysis described, systematic and rigorous? Are competing arguments presented?
14 *Was the study design flexible and responsive?*	Findings should be used to generate plans and ideas for change and be flexible in the light of real-world issues.

Question	Explanation
15 *Are there clear statements of the findings and outcomes of each phase of the study?*	Findings and outcomes should be presented clearly, logically and explicitly for each phase of the study. They should be discussed critically.
16 *Do the researchers link the data that are presented to their own commentary and interpretation?*	There should be a discussion of how participants were engaged in reflection and the methods used, with a clear distinction made between data and interpretation. Researchers should critically examine their own and others' roles in the interpretation of data.
17 *Is there discussion of the extent to which aims and objectives were achieved at each stage?*	It should be clear as to whether the action research objectives have been met, and the reasons for successes and failures analysed.
18 *Are the findings of the study transferable?*	The context of the study should be clearly described so that a judgement can be made by readers concerning the transferability of the findings to other settings.
19 *Have the authors articulated the criteria upon which their own work is to be read/judged?*	Authors should justify the perspective from which the proposal or report should be interpreted.

Critical analysis of action research studies

• • • REFLECTIVE ACTIVITY 10.3 • • •

In order to demonstrate the usefulness of different methods of critiquing action research studies, undertake the following exercises, looking at three different papers from around the world using the ideas presented above. A contemporary way of accessing the recommended papers is to cut and paste the DOI (Digital Object Identifier, used for online publishing; see http://www.doi.org/) into your web browser. If this does not get you free full-text access, you will need to use the search engines from your university or NHS Hospital Trust to search for the papers, or try using NHS Evidence (which is a free-to-use NHS search engine at www.evidence.nhs.uk).

1 Find the following paper: Vallenga, D, Grypdonck, MHF, Tan, FIY, Lendemeijer, BHGM and Boon, PAJM (2008) Improving decision-making in caring for people with epilepsy and intellectual disability: an action research project. *Journal of Advanced Nursing* 61(3): 261–272. DOI: 10.1111/j.1365-2648.2007.04477.x.

Using Waterman et al.'s (2001) 20 questions, work through the paper and come to an overall assessment of its quality.

2 Find the following paper: Nomura, M, Makimoto, K, Kato, M, Shiba, T, Matsuura, C, Shigenobu, K, Ishikawa, T, Matsumoto, N and Ikeda, M (2009) Empowering older people with early dementia and family caregivers: A participatory action research study. *International Journal of Nursing Studies* 46: 431–441.DOI: 10.1016/j.ijnurstu.2007.09.009.

Using Bradbury and Reason's (2006) criteria, work through the paper and come to an overall assessment of its quality.

3 Find the following paper: Dickson, G (2000) Aboriginal grandmothers' experience with health promotion and participatory action research. *Qualitative Health Research* 10: 188–213. DOI: 10.1177/104973200129118363.

Using Gomm et al.'s (2001) criteria, work through the paper and come to an overall assessment of its quality.

An assessment of the quality of the paper by Vallenga et al. (2008), using Waterman et al.'s (2001) 20 questions is provided in the commentary that has been added to Table 10.5a (see Table 10.5b). Overall, this is a well-written paper which gives a good deal of information about what seems to be a rigorously-conducted study. There is a clear commitment to improving decision making and empowering clients. One limitation is the exclusion of clients from the study, but this is argued and justified by the authors and their arguments are logical. Client relatives are included instead, but have not participated as fully as staff. Naming the location as Kempenhaeghe is worrying as it identifies clients to people who are outside the research study.

An assessment of quality of the paper by Nomura et al. (2009) using Bradbury and Reason's (2006) criteria is provided in Table 10.4b. Overall, this seems to be a well-written paper which is informative and appears to have made a real difference to their client group. There is prolonged engagement in the setting and enough contextual and procedural data for readers to make their own judgement as to the transferability of the study. The paper has very limited information about ethical issues other than to say that permission was granted by the local ethics committee. There is no discussion of confidentiality, anonymity, informed consent or rights to withdraw that would be usual in other research studies. If used as an 'assessment tool', as Bradbury and Reason's work does not explicitly take ethical issues into account, it would 'miss' the research ethics dimension of studies. It may be that in Japan there are cultural issues, or that their participants had medical issues meaning that informed consent was not possible, although as they are described as having early dementia this is not clear. In the UK, the Mental Capacity Act 2005 (Department of Health 2005) means

Table 10.5b 20 questions for judging the rigour of action research with commentary (adapted from Waterman et al. 2001)

Question	Explanation	Commentary
1 *Are the aims and objectives of each stage of the research clearly stated?*	Did the authors of the project clearly define the aims and objectives of the project and were they appropriate?	On p. 262 there is a clear statement of research questions and aims, concerning improving decision making and empowerment.
2 *Was the action research relevant to practitioners and/or users?*	Action research should: address local issues; contribute to new understanding; be relevant to participants; suggest further research and make recommendations for policy and practice	The field is outlined and appears highly relevant.
3 **Were the phases of the project clearly outlined?*	Was a logical process in evidence (or intended)? Should include: • problem identification • planning • action • evaluation.	Figures 1, 3 & 6 and Table 1 give good outlines of the project stages.
4 **Were the participants and stakeholders clearly described and justified?*	Did the project focus on service users and/or health professionals? How were participants selected and recruited for each phase of the project?	Staff and relatives were involved in the action research project but clients were not as most were held not capable of fully understanding the issues and processes. Relatives did not participate face-to-face as fully as staff.
5 **Was consideration given to the local context while implementing change?*	Contextual factors should be discussed, such as why it was selected, and a critical examination of values, beliefs and power relationships should be included.	There is a good background section and also the local context is well described in Figure 2.
6 **Was the relationship between researchers and participants adequately considered?*	The level and extent of participation should be clearly defined for each stage; there should be reflexivity by all involved.	Some mention of reflection. The relationship has been considered but it is not an 'equal' one as the authors argue that clients mostly were not really capable of active participation.

(Continued)

Table 10.5b *(Continued)*

Question	Explanation	Commentary
7 *Was the project managed appropriately?*	Key persons in organisations should have been involved; those involved need requisite skills to implement change and/or research; implementation plans should be feasible, achievable, and clearly a result of local participation.	It's not entirely clear the extent to which this study meets these criteria, but all clinical staff groups seem to be represented. Management initiated the study.
8 *Were ethical issues encountered and how were they dealt with?*	Rights of participants, researchers and those affected by the action research process all require consideration, including confidentiality and informed consent.	Some ethical issues have been addressed and there is a clear statement of ethics approval in the section on p. 265. The location is named as Kempenhaeghe in the acknowledgements.
9 *Was the study adequately funded/supported?*	Were the assessments of cost and resources realistic? Were there any conflicts of interest?	Not discussed.
10 *Was the length and timetable of the project realistic?*	Was the project completed on time? Was there slippage of the timeline?	The project seems to have been open-ended. 'Ruby Road' ran over 2 years; 'Agate Lane' over 18 months.
11 *Were data collected in a way that addressed the research issue?*	Were appropriate research methodologies, methods of data collection and analysis used to answer research questions?	Data were collected using focus groups, questionnaires, observation and 'written documents'. The lead researcher kept a personal reflective diary.
12 *Were steps taken to promote the rigour of the findings?*	Differing perspectives on issues should be used, as should method, glossary and theoretical triangulation. Key findings should be fed back to participants and their feedback used. Reflexive accounts should be offered.	A strength of this paper is that multi-method triangulation was undertaken, with some input from an external researcher. There seems to have been a real process of reflection and discussion with staff, although there does not seem to be any explicit section of 'reflective accounts'.
13 *Were data analyses sufficiently rigorous?*	Were procedures for analysis described, systematic and rigorous? Are competing arguments presented?	Verbatim transcripts and data from each action cycle were structured thematically and analysed using the constant comparative method. Not clear the extent to which competing perspectives are presented.

Table 10.5b ***(Continued)***

Question	Explanation	Commentary
14 *Was the study design flexible and responsive?*	Findings should be used to generate plans and ideas for change and be flexible in the light of real-world issues.	Ruby Road and Agate Lane both followed different paths and it seems as if the cycles and discussions were flexible and centred on real-world concerns.
15 *Are there clear statements of the findings and outcomes of each phase of the study?*	Findings and outcomes should be presented clearly, logically and explicitly for each phase of the study. They should be discussed critically.	Difficult to do this in a single journal article with multiple action cycles over 18 months & 2 years. The overall summaries are good per location. Key findings are discussed as resulting from work in particular phases.
16 *Do the researchers link the data that are presented to their own commentary and interpretation?*	There should be a discussion of how participants were engaged in reflection and the methods used, with a clear distinction made between data and interpretation. Researchers should critically examine their own and others' roles in the interpretation of data.	No clear statement about methods of reflection. Some mention of influence of self and others' interpretations. Findings clearly relate to work undertaken in each location and different phases.
18 *Is there discussion of the extent to which aims and objectives were achieved at each stage?*	It should be clear as to whether the action research objectives have been met, and the reasons for successes and failures analysed.	The discussion section gives an overall assessment of this and there is some discussion of the way in which discussion led to particular outcomes in the findings section.
19 *Are the findings of the study transferable?*	The context of the study should be clearly described so that a judgement can be made by readers concerning the transferability of the findings to other settings.	They argue that transferability cannot be empirically substantiated but there is enough context and detail for readers to make informed judgements about the study and its relevance to their own settings.
20 *Have the authors articulated the criteria upon which their own work is to be read/judged?*	Authors should justify the perspective from which the proposal or report should be interpreted.	They talk about the rigorous application of a pragmatic, cyclical approach, methodological and researcher triangulation as steps to reinforce validity. These were met.

Table 10.4b Issues as choice-points and questions for quality in action research (adapted from Bradbury and Reason 2006: 350)

- **Explicit development of praxis and participation**

  Improving the situation for their participants is explicit throughout the study. They used a participatory action research approach to develop a group activity programme for community-dwelling elderly people with early dementia and counselling programmes for family caregivers. The main focus was with caregivers, who were part of a focus group and counselling services, and data from persons with dementia (PsWD) were included to monitor any changes in activity and behaviour. Additional data were also collected by caregivers' observations of their PWD. The study operated at individual, group and community level.

- **Guided by concern for outcomes**

  Arguably, there is a strong concern for outcomes, particularly the empowerment of the PsWD. The word 'empower' is used 25 times in the text and is central to the whole paper.

- **Includes a variety of forms of investigation**

  Data were collected in various ways: observational data were collected during activities, written comments from the caregivers, phone interviews and counselling with caregivers. A portfolio for each PWD and caregiver was constructed for analysis.

- **Worthy of the term 'significant'**

  This study lasted for five years and included three cycles: individual, group and community. The first cycle involved intervention to regain procedural skills for each PWD through a cooking programme. The second cycle increased interactions with family members and other PsWD through group activities that promoted communication and visits to temples and shrines. The third cycle fostered community participation through culturally relevant activities. PsWD demonstrated their skills and regained confidence. For family caregivers, the programme provided knowledge about dementia and the utilisation of social resources. Counselling offered coaching on problem-focused coping and helped caregivers to recognise the symptoms of dementia and reduce behavioural problems. Overall, cognitive rehabilitation helped restore lost skills and confidence for PsWD, illustrating the importance of interventions for community-dwelling elderly with early dementia and their families. These do seem to be 'significant' outcomes.

- **Developing new infrastructures for working practices**

  New infrastructures and working practices were established. When the project became more widely recognised, they received many new referrals. There was already a good social network in this small rural town. What is not clear is the extent to which these structures endured after the project ended.

that everyone is taken to have the capacity to consent unless it is demonstrated otherwise.This would make obtaining consent in this study a legal requirement.

An assessment of the quality of the paper by Dickson (2000) using Gomm et al.'s (2001) criteria is presented in Table 10.3b. This schedule of questions seems to focus on the credibility of the research, and this focus makes Dickson's (2000) paper look questionable as there is, arguably, a lack of perspective and balance on the part of the writer, who has collected and analysed all the data, is very close to the participants and presents the work in a highly favourable light. While these are valid criticisms of action research

Table 10.3b Gomm et al.'s questions for evaluating the quality of action research with commentary (adapted from Gomm et al. 2000)

Questions	Issues	Commentary
1 **Evidence of change**		
Is there evidence that the action has taken place because of the 'intervention'? How has the situation before and after the study been described? Are effects for all those involved discussed?	What measures or criteria have been used to demonstrate the research claims? Is testimonial evidence reliable? Or is there a one-sided perspective which only shows the project in a good light?	There is evidence of change in that attitudes and behaviour of the grandmothers is reported to have changed as a result of their increased confidence and understanding. These are not measured as such. Some evidence is presented in the form of quotes. It is not possible to say what the benefits for each individual are, but culturally the collective benefits are more important than the individual ones for this study. There is little critical material on the study.
2 **Replicability**		
Could a similar project be undertaken elsewhere? Including • What was done? • Characteristics of all those involved • Resourcing • Local context	As action research involves complex change scenarios, is enough detail included for readers to judge the extent of transferability?	The study comprised a series of weekly meetings with the broad premise of bringing together aboriginal women for support. This is not in itself complex, but the material presented does indicate a richness and complexity, rooted in the grandmothers' culture. A similar project could be undertaken elsewhere, and while the schedule of meetings could be easily achieved, the discussions and outcomes for participants would be entirely different.
3 **'Experiment effect'**		
Is it clear how much the intervention and/or how much the energy and enthusiasm of those involved contributed to the change?	Enthusiasm may be enough; an effective change strategy would be needed for transferability.	Any changes resulting from the project seem clearly to come from the grandmothers and their shared sense of community and support. However, this would not have been developed without the researcher's facilitation and enthusiasm.

(Continued)

Table 10.3b *(Continued)*

Questions	Issues	Commentary
4. **Biased reporting**		
How likely is it that the report was written to give the project a favourable light?	As collaborative projects, action research reports are likely to represent consensus between participants, and may not represent the full story.	There is little or no attempt to report conflicting perspectives from within this project and the author has a strong interest in presenting the study in a favourable light as it was her PhD. Indeed, there are some contradictory ideas in the paper which go unremarked. For example, both aboriginal culture and Canadian society are described as patriarchical and oppressive towards women: as a theme of the study was to 'connect with the self', which included cultural and spiritual identity, then, arguably, fostering a white-western individualistic persona for these grandmothers may conflict with their traditional understanding of themselves, and may be seen as imposing the author's feminist-inspired ideas on them.
5. **Insight and understanding**		
How much of each are proffered which may improve practice elsewhere?	Is there clear transferability?	There is a lot of insight and understating offered into the lives and worlds of these grandmothers. There is a lot of contextual and cultural information given which makes the study rich and interesting to read. It is widely transferable in the sense that the structure of regular group meetings is easy to achieve. Other cultural aspects of the study mean that it is highly specific to time and location, and it is therefore described by the author as a case study.

and should not be dismissed, focusing on them misses some of the apparently positive aspects of this study, which fostered well-being and a sense of community support among these grandmothers, ending their isolation and connecting them to the wider social and political world. It is a well-written and engaging paper and the study appears to have helped the participants cope with their lives. It does raise questions concerning the imposition of some western values on the aboriginal women and also does not have a clearly-structured cyclical methodology, as do the other two papers critiqued above.

Critical evaluation

There are certain similarities between these authors' ideas on the quality of action research, and their work has similarities in the broad areas listed in Table 10.6.

Although this is a very broad level of analysis of key authors' view on 'quality' in AR, we conclude that the key issues to be addressed in action research reports are that they:

- generate new knowledge;
- produce change;
- have an ethic of participation;
- demonstrate rigorous methods of inquiry; and are
- transferable (meaning that they make sense to others in different settings).

There are several areas where the authors' views have differences in emphasis: Herr and Anderson (2005) and Gomm et al. (2000) have an explicit view about the necessity of change, but this is not so explicit for Koch and Kralik (2006). Also, only Waterman et al. (2001) make it explicit that ethical issues should be made clear and discussed, although an ethical dimension is an element of all the authors' work in the sense that fostering participation in AR is an ethical issue in itself. In critically appraising the frameworks themselves rather than simply the data they contain, it is an obvious point but one worth making, that while they are reasonably detailed, they can never fully do justice to the complexity and context-bound nature of an action research study (Bradbury and Reason 2006; Koch and Kralik 2006) and so must be viewed as taking a 'broad brush' approach to the evaluation of action research work. The question for readers to decide for themselves, and this chapter has helped you work towards your own answer, is whether this inability to do justice to each individual action research study is worth the compromise in providing common ground for the stakeholders we identified earlier.

Table 10.6 Key areas of similarity in authors' ideas of evaluating the quality of action research

Areas of similarity	Authors
Generates new knowledge	Herr and Anderson (2005) Gomm et al. (2000)
Produces change	Herr and Anderson (2005) Gomm et al. (2000) Bradbury and Reason (2006) Waterman et al. (2001)
An ethic of participation	Koch and Kralik (2006) Coghlan and Brannick (2010) Bradbury and Reason (2006) Waterman et al. (2001)
Demonstration of rigorous methods	Koch and Kralik (2006) Waterman et al. (2001)
Transferability	Gomm et al. (2000) Waterman et al. (2001) Koch and Kralik (2006)

Summary

Some authors argue that evaluative criteria are not required in action research as each study is unique and stands and falls on its own context and description. However, arguably, it seems reasonable that stakeholders need a shared understanding of the quality of action research proposals and reports. There are many ideas about judging the quality of action research and this chapter has listed six of them, and allowed the reader to explore how they might be used to critique AR reports, and where key similarities and differences lie.

Further reading

Dick, B (2000) *A beginner's guide to action research* [Online]. Available at: www.scu.edu.au/schools/gcm/ar/arp/guide.html (accessed 6/11/2009). Describes action research and its simultaneous achievement of change and research.

Karim, K (2001) Assessing the strengths and weaknesses of action research. *Nursing Standard* 15(26): 33–35. Useful short summary of some relevant literature.

Meyer, J (2000) Evaluating action research. *Age and Ageing* 29(S2): 8–10. Available online at: http://ageing.oxfordjournals.org/cgi/reprint/29/suppl_2/8.pdf (accessed 6/11/2009). Argues that action research is relevant to practice because of the central involvement of participants.

Piggot-Irvine, E and Bartlett, B (2008) *Evaluating action research*. Wellington. New Zealand: Centre for Educational Research. Seeks to answer questions about the value and quality of an action research project, and the value and quality that should be expected.

Useful websites

AGREE Collaboration website, Appraisal of Guidelines Research and Appraisal: www.agreecollaboration.org/instrument/ has a tool using criteria that also gives a numerical scoring system.

CAENTI (Coordination Action of the European Network for Territorial Intelligence): www.territorial-intelligence.eu/caenti/quality/ focuses on sustainable development, with a tool for assessing related action research studies.

CASP, the NHS Public Health Research Unit Critical Appraisal Skills Programme: www.phru.nhs.uk/pages/PHD/CASP.htm provides criteria-based tools for evaluating all types of research and systematic reviews.

Collaborative, participatory and empowerment evaluation. Website of the American Evaluation Association topical interest group. The American Evaluation Association's mission is to extend and improve evaluation practices and methods, and support the generation of theory and knowledge about effective human action. http://homepage.mac.com/profdavidf/empowermentevaluation.htm provides some useful resources, including books and publications, tools and guides.

References

Bradbury, H and Reason, P (2006) Broadening the bandwidth of validity: Issues and choice-points for improving the quality of action research. In P Reason and H Bradbury (eds), *Handbook of action research* (2nd edition). London: Sage, Chapter 33.

Coghlan, D and Brannick, T (2010) *Doing action research in your own organisation* (3rd edition). London: Sage.

Department of Health (2005) Mental Capacity Act. Available online at: www.dh.gov.uk/en/SocialCare/Deliveringadultsocialcare/MentalCapacity/MentalCapacityAct2005/index.htm (accessed 3/11/2009).

Dickson, G (2000) Aboriginal grandmothers' experience with health promotion and participatory action research. *Qualitative Health Research* 10: 188–213.DOI: 10.1177/104973200129118363.

Elliott, J (2007) Assessing the quality of action research. *Research Papers in Education* 22(2): 229–246.

Gomm, R, Needham, G and Bullman, A (2000) *Evaluating research in health and social care*. London: Sage.

Guba, E and Libcoln, Y (1989) *Fourth generation evaluation*. Thousand Oaks, CA: Sage.

Herr, K and Anderson, G L (2005) *The action research dissertation: A guide for students and faculty*. London: Sage.

Koch, T and Kralik, D (2006) *Participatory action research in healthcare*. Oxford: Blackwell.

Nomura, M, Makimoto, K, Kato, M, Shiba, T, Matsuura, C, Shigenobu, K, Ishikawa, T, Matsumoto, N and Ikeda, M (2009) Empowering older people with early dementia and family caregivers: A participatory action research study. *International Journal of Nursing Studies* 46: 431–441. DOI: 10.1016/j.ijnurstu.2007.09.009.

Stake, R E and Schwandt, T A (2006) On discerning quality in evaluation. In I Shaw, M Mark and J Greene (eds), *Handbook of evaluation*. New York: Sage.

Vallenga, D, Grypdonck, M H F, Tan, F I Y, Lendemeijer, B H G M and Boon, P A J M (2008) Improving decision-making in caring for people with epilepsy and intellectual disability: An action research project. *Journal of Advanced Nursing* 61(3): 261–272.

Waterman, H, Tillen, D, Dickson, R and de Koning, K (2001) Action research: A systematic review and guidance for assessment. *Health Technology Assessment* 5(23): 1–166. Southampton: The National Coordinating Centre for Health Technology Assessment. Available online at: www.ncchta.org/project/1007.asp (accessed 29/6/2011).

CONCLUSIONS

LOOKING TO THE FUTURE

Modern healthcare practice, with its focus on continuous change, innovation and efficiency, requires a contemporary research approach to advance patient care in clinical settings and organisations that are constantly changing and evolving. Action research symbolises much of what modern research should be about – analysing the world but also trying to change it (Gray 2009) in complex settings and contexts that are frequently less than ideal. Action research is used withinclinical practice, practitioner research, practice development, applied research and knowledge transfer. The methodology also sits within the umbrella term of implementation science. In the future, to make a difference to patients and to advance the science, researchers will need to recognise, grapple with and not ignore the messy, complex and frequent uncertainty of clinical practice settings (Rycroft-Malone and Burton 2010). The four sections of this book have attempted to provide a contemporary understanding of action research for healthcare settings through its origins and development, the challenges, costs and benefits of using the methodology, and ways of evaluating and communicating the process and outcomes of the approach.

Within the 'What is Action Research?' section, it is evident that action research has, in comparison to traditional research approaches, a relatively short history which is surrounded by controversy that remains to this day. The focus of Kurt Lewin's early action research in the 1940s was to solve social problems. Over the past two decades the methodology has often been subsumed within the critical paradigm. Critical studies take the research process to the people who are experiencing the phenomenon and assume that knowledge generation is a political activity (Fontana 2004). For the future, critical studies seem a logical fit for healthcare and nursing's commitment to society:

> Caring and critical seem, on the surface, to be at odds with one another but in nursing practice they are inseparable. While nurses and health care practitioners deliver care, they critique the health of their patients contextually and encourage patient involvement and participation with the intent of empowerment and health. They look for contradiction in what is happening to the patient and use reflection to evaluate their ability to improve care. (Fontana 2004: 100)

The 'Why Choose Action Research?' section seems self-evident for a healthcare practitioner wishing to adopt this systematic approach for change and development in clinical practice. The action research approach is akin to the stages of the nursing process, with a central focus on critique of, and reflection on, practice leading to change. Increasing knowledge of the research process and use of the methodology enables recognition of, and an ability to continuously develop, contemporary healthcare knowledge, including creative and advanced practice skills. The skills include political acumen and leadership, collaborative practice with stakeholders, including patients, their supporters and other members of the multi-professional team, participative facilitation as well as enhancing personal insight and self-awareness. The critical thinking skills that develop lead to critical knowing and, as Fontana (2004) suggests, can be introduced to students and used as an additional fundamental pattern of knowing in nursing.

The chapters in the 'Conducting Action Research in Clinical Practice' section have built on the content of the previous two sections. While every action research project is unique, the personal account of a Consultant Nurse and the subsequent chapter on collaborative working in complex clinical settings provide significant insight into the clinical action research process in the real-world context. The ethical considerations chapter provides a contemporary perspective on, in particular, the nature of action research in regard to anonymity/confidentiality and informed consent. There are still many gaps in knowledge, in particular much more needs to be documented on engaging and supporting patients and carers in clinical action research studies, including appropriate ways of obtaining ethical clearance and the impact of collaboration, joint working and learning leading to 'action'.

Ways of sharing the process and outcomes of clinical action research have been developed within the section entitled 'Disseminating and Evaluating Clinical Action Research Projects'. The importance of writing clinical action research within different medium and its presentation to diverse audiences demonstrates the need for us all to continue to develop our writing and presentation skills and share the methodology, and the findings from our projects, with a wide audience. In the final chapter we hope that different ways of making judgements about clinical action research projects and ways of evaluating the research process and outcome will support the understanding of many more studies in the future.

Future UK perspective

Action research is a contemporary research approach that can support the UK's vision of nursing and healthcare for the twenty-first century in delivering high-quality, compassionate care, integrating research evidence into clinical practice, and leading clinical change and innovation. The methodology reflects an approach which integrates practice, education and research. As has been argued in this text (in Chapters 4 and 6), there is an overwhelming UK-wide need for increasing clinical academic integration.

For England:

> Urgent steps must be taken to strengthen the integration of nursing and midwifery practice, education and research; develop and sustain the educational workforce; facilitate sustainable clinical academic career pathways; and further develop nurses' and midwives' research skills. (Department of Health 2010: 7)

For Scotland:

> Boundaries between education and practice will blur as education becomes increasingly recognised as being pivotal to best practice and as individuals move between academic and practice settings in the context of new organisational partnerships. ... Academic, research and clinical academic careers must be developed and sustained to ensure the best learning and development opportunities for future nursing and midwifery students and practitioners. The role and value of educators will continue to evolve from that of knowledge-provider to facilitator of knowledge acquisition and utilisation. (NHS Education for Scotland, 2009: 2)

For Northern Ireland: within the theme Improving Outcomes through Innovation –

- Nurses, midwives and support staff will identify opportunities for practice/service improvements and communicate these to line managers.
- Nurses, midwives and support staff will spread and embed innovation *and research findings to improve outcomes for patients and clients.* (Department of Health, Social Services and Public Safety 2010: 11)

For Wales:

> Employer organisations (Service Providers and Higher Education Institutions) should consider introducing a 'revolving door' model, which enables staff to move between service and education/research settings. ... Employer organisations develop clinical academic posts to undertake and facilitate the expansion of clinically based programmes of research, linked to the research activities within Higher Education Institutes. ...Senior Lecturing/Research staff employed in academic posts receive support to develop expertise in teaching and develop a research portfolio, which includes receiving coaching and supervision from more experienced researchers. (Welsh Assembly Government 2009: 21). This will also help to enhance research supervision of action research projects (see Chapter 7).

The above proposals clearly demonstrate the need to integrate practice, education and research across the UK. Recognition of clinical academic collaboration will benefit patients and students as well as clinical and academic staff. One proposed way, demonstrated throughout this book, is by sharing knowledge and skills and working and learning together within a clinical action research project.

In the UK, the mission of the Academy for Nursing, Midwifery and Health Visiting is to play an active part in maximising research for patient benefit and enhancing the return of the public's investment in health-related research. The Academy is an amalgamation of leading healthcare organisations and its prime concern is to be:

> an expert collaborative voice for all aspects of research involving nursing, midwifery and health visiting in the UK, including policy development, its implementation and evaluation, through negotiation and dialogue with other key stakeholders. (Academy of Nursing, Midwifery and Health Visiting UK, undated)

One of the key themes of the Academy is 'Service and Research'. Recognition and action are required now and in the future to support a clinical academic culture in healthcare organisations, with a focus on valuing and enabling practice-based research and development for patient benefit. There is growing strategic recognition of the need for clinical chairs and joint appointments (Girot 2010). Further ways to accomplish *clinical* academic research development include: devising creative degree pathways encompassing clinical action research, and accredited work-based learning programmes for participating in a clinical action research project. Our past, current and future perspective for the UK is encompassed within the assertion by a New Zealand lecturer:

> I believe that action research should be the mainstay of nursing research activity. It is still in its infancy in our profession, but I would like to see its use dramatically escalate over the coming decade. Extensive use of action research is likely to facilitate the move away from introspective 'navel-gazing' nursing research that offers little by way of tangible practice-orientated change and outcomes ... (Whitehead 2005: 1032)

A global snapshot of action research

We thought it would be interesting to gain a global 'snapshot' of the extent to which action research has recently been used, to give us an indication of the diversity of action research, and also inform thinking in regard to knowledge gaps for future projects. We addressed the question: What issues are being discussed globally in AR in healthcare practice?

A literature search was conducted in May 2009 in specific journals chosen for their scope, relevance and English-language publication. Most are international journals, but the journals *American Journal of Nursing, Australian Journal of Advanced Nursing* and *Scandinavian Journal of Caring Sciences* were all chosen to explore areas that were not represented in the international journals. The search parameters from 2000 to 2009 reflect contemporary trends in global AR publishing. All studies retrieved for the snapshot report empirical research rather than literature reviews, opinion pieces or methodological discussions. Where journals have returned no hits, this information has been included to show that the journal was searched. The search results are presented in Table 11.1.

This search process identified a total of 50 papers for review, and these were grouped into the geographical areas indicated in Table 11.2, including the number of papers retrieved in each area, themes from each geographical area and the papers exhibiting characteristics for each theme. The themes represent the major focus of the paper, so for example, while PAR is an approach to doing AR and other papers use other approaches, PAR is included as a theme because authors have specifically used this terminology to describe their study design, whereas other authors have used a wide variety of more generic terminology. Other themes reflect the field in which the authors were working, so that improving clinical care or health education are more central aspects. Papers can appear in more than one theme, so that both PAR and health promotion may be important features. Themes are different in different geographical locations due to their different usages in those.

Australia, New Zealand and the rest of the world

Four key areas were evident concerning action research literature published in the chosen journals in Australia, New Zealand and the rest of the world. Papers from the rest of the world included one each from United Arab Emirates, Thailand, an African study in 37 counties, Japan and Guatemala. Of the 14 papers retrieved, six utilised frameworks based on participatory action research (PAR) (Busza 2004; Day et al. 2009; de la Rue 2003; Koch and Kralik 2008; Liza and Elsom 2008; Nomura et al. 2009). This has an explicitly emancipatory focus which emphasises the political potential of the work. The other eight described themselves as action research studies (Brumley et al. 2006; Buskens 2008; Dickson 2008; Heslop et al. 2000; Khresheh and Barclay 2007; McAllister and Stockhausen 2001; Mills and Fitzgerald 2008; Wai-tong et al. 2002), of which one (Buskens 2008) uses the term 'emancipatory'. There were a variety of areas addressed, but seven were dedicated to improving clinical care by direct or indirect means, such as service or knowledge improvement among clinical staff (Brumley et al. 2006; Busza 2004; Day et al. 2009; Heslop et al. 2000; Khresheh and Barclay 2007; Mills and Fitzgerald 2008; Nomura et al. 2009). Four papers were dedicated to improving health more broadly in community settings (Buskens 2008; Day et al. 2009; Dickson 2008; Koch and Kralik 2008). The focus of four studies was improving aspects of healthcare education (de la Rue 2003; McAllister and Stockhausen 2001; Wai-tong et al. 2002).

Table 11.1 Snapshot literature search

Journal title	Journal relevance	Search terms	Number of hits	Inclusion criteria	Number of empirical research papers retrieved
International Journal of Nursing Studies	Peer review international nursing journal	Action and research as title word or sentence	1481	Research studies published between 2000 and 2009, relevant to healthcare	6
Journal of Advanced Nursing	Peer review international nursing journal	Action and research as title word or sentence	21	Research studies published between 2000 and 2009, relevant to healthcare	11
Qualitative Health Research	Peer review international, interdisciplinary research journal	Action and research as title word or sentence	10	Research studies published between 2000 and 2009, relevant to healthcare	6
Action Research	Peer review international, interdisciplinary research journal	1. Action and research as title word or sentence	83	Research studies published between 2000 and 2009, relevant to healthcare	8
		2. Health as key word	70		7
Action Research International	Peer review international, interdisciplinary research journal (online)	All articles scrutinised	0	No relevant research studies published between 2000 and 2009, relevant to healthcare	0
Educational Action Research	Peer review international, interdisciplinary research journal	1. Health as key word 2. Nursing as key word	86 5	Research studies published between 2000 and 2009, relevant to healthcare	7 0
International Journal of Action Research	Peer review international, interdisciplinary research journal	All articles scrutinised	0	Research studies published between 2000 and 2009, relevant to healthcare	0
American Journal of Nursing	Nurses' journal from the USA with a wide readership	Action and research as title word or sentence	0	Research studies published between 2000 and 2009, relevant to healthcare	0
Australian Journal of Advanced Nursing	Australian research journal	Action and research as title word or sentence	31	Research studies published between 2000 and 2009, relevant to healthcare	4
Scandinavian Journal of Caring Sciences		Action research as key words	363	Research studies published between 2000 and 2009, relevant to healthcare	1

Table 11.2 Themes from the literature based on geographical area

Geographical area	Number of papers retrieved	Themes	Papers in each theme
Australia, New Zealand and the rest of the world	14	Participatory action research	*de la Rue (2003); *Busza (2004); *Day et al. (2009); *Nomura et al. (2009); Liza and Elsom (2008); Koch and Kralik (2008).
		Improving clinical care	*Busza (2004); Brumley et al. (2006); *Day et al. (2009); Heslop et al. (2000); Khresheh and Barclay (2007); Mills and Fitzgerald (2008); *Nomura et al. (2009).
		Improving healthcare education	Wai-tong et al. (2002); McAllister and Stockhausen (2001); *de la Rue (2003).
		Improving community health	Buskens (2008); *Day et al. (2009); Dickson, G (2008); Koch and Kralik (2008).
Europe	9	Participatory action research	*Iversen et al. (2006); Poulsen et al. (2007); *Vallenga et al. (2008).
		Health promotion	Jacobs (2006); *Iversen et al. (2006); Philips ME (2004).
		Improving clinical care	Beukema and Valkenburg (2007); Portillo et al. (2009); *Vallenga et al. (2008); Vatne et al. (2009).
United Kingdom and Ireland	16	Participatory action research	*Chiu (2003); *Stuttaford and Coe (2007).
		Health promotion	*Chiu (2003); Kilgour and Fleming (2001); Neuls (2003); Lavie-Ajayi et al. (2007).
		Organisational change	Bridges et al. (2003); Bridges and Meyer (2007); Cooper and Hewison (2002); Elsey and Lathlean (2006); Kelly and Simpson (2008); Kemp (2000); *Stuttaford and Coe (2007); Waterman et al. (2007); Williamson and Prosser (2002); Williamson et al. (2004).
		Improving clinical care	Waterman et al. (2005a); Waterman et al. (2005b); Stead et al. (2001).
United States and Canada	11	Participatory action research	*Baker and Wang (2006); *Choudhry et al. (2004); *Flicker et al. (2008); *Reid et al. (2006); *Lind (2007); *Maiter et al. (2008); *Mendenhall and Doherty (2007); *Teram et al. (2005); *Westhues et al. (2008).
		Health promotion	Amsden and VanWynsberghe (2005); *Baker and Wang (2006); *Choudhry et al. (2004); *Flicker et al. (2008); *Reid et al. (2006); *Lind (2007); *Maiter et al. (2008); *Mendenhall and Doherty (2007); Nelson et al.(2004); *Teram et al. (2005); *Westhues et al. (2008).
	Total = 50		*Paper appears in more than one theme

Europe

Again, in the European papers, PAR methods were used but not so extensively as in Australia, New Zealand and the rest of the world with 3/9 reporting this approach (Iversen et al. 2006; Poulsen et al. 2007; Vallenga et al. 2008). Three studies (Iversen et al. 2006; Jacobs 2006; Philips 2004) had as their subject health promotion in the sense of improving or empowering participants to improve their health, while a further four studies (Beukema and Valkenburg 2007; Portillo et al. 2009; Vallenga et al. 2008; Vatne et al. 2009) were concerned with improving clinical care by introducing or improving aspects of care delivery for patients and clients.

UK and Ireland

The focus of action research papers in the UK and Ireland was different from that elsewhere in the world. There were only two (Chiu 2003; Stuttaford and Coe 2007) with avowedly PAR methodologies, with others more generally stating they used action research. While four focused on health promotion (Chiu 2003; Kilgour and Fleming 2001); Lavie-Ajayi et al. 2007; Neuls 2003) and three on improving clinical care (Waterman et al. 2005a; Waterman et al. 2005b; Stead et al. 2001), the majority of papers (10/16) were concerned with organisational change (Bridges et al. 2003; Bridges and Meyer 2007; Cooper and Hewison 2002; Elsey and Lathlean 2006; Kelly and Simpson 2008; Kemp 2000; Stuttaford and Coe 2007; Waterman et al 2007; Williamson and Prosser 2002; Williamson et al. 2004), that is, developing some aspect of the ways in which organisations worked in order to improve outcomes for that organisation and for its staff. There may have been beneficial outcomes for patients and clients in this organisational development, but these were not the primary motivation for the studies. Thus, according to the findings from these selected journals, action research is taking place in healthcare settings in the UK, but is not perhaps so well focused on or translated directly into improvement in clinical care or patient/client outcomes as it is towards organisational development.

USA and Canada

The focus from North America was entirely on health promotion, no other areas featured in this snapshot review, and 11 studies were retrieved (Amsden and VanWynsberghe 2005; Baker and Wang 2006; Choudhry et al. 2004;

Flicker et al. 2008; Lind 2007; Maiter et al. 2008; Mendenhall and Doherty 2007; Nelson et al. 2004; Reid et al. 2006; Teram et al. 2005; Westhues et al. 2008). Nine of the 11 studies retrieved used PAR methodologies (Baker and Wang 2006; Choudhry et al. 2004; Flicker et al. 2008; Lind 2007; Maiter et al. 2008; Mendenhall and Doherty 2007; Reid et al. 2006; Teram et al. 2005; Westhues et al. 2008), indicating that this action research approach appears to currently be popular in North America.

Evaluation

This review serves as a 'snapshot' of the literature published in journals selected for their international healthcare scope and relevance. It gives a global perspective on action research work, although it does not take into account unpublished studies or studies that might be published in smaller, national journals. It is thus acknowledged as being limited. However, some key points are evident:

- Health promotion appears to be a major focus of global action research.
- PAR currently appears to be a popular approach, particularly in North America, Australia and New Zealand, but less so in the UK and Ireland.
- Improving clinical care appears to be a feature of global action research, except in the UK and Ireland where the overwhelming feature is organisational change.

Final thoughts

The need to develop an understanding of clinical action research is evident and is of particular relevance as we enter a time of immense change within the UK healthcare system. We anticipate that the use of action research in healthcare settings will continue to increase across the globe as research cannot sit separately to the real-world context in which healthcare practitioners work and patients receive care. We hope that this book has helped to support and increase understanding of what we believe is essential knowledge for healthcare practitioners and academic colleagues. We recognise that we may not have met all the needs of interested practitioners and colleagues but see this book as a practical and complementary text to the current action research literature.

There is much to consider regarding the successful undertaking of this approach, including linking clinical change and development projects with local healthcare policy for quality and service improvement. When conducting your project always remember *three essential points*: (1) others (who went on to successfully complete their project) will have experienced similar challenges along the way; (2) throughout the research journey ensure appropriate, ongoing support for yourself and the co-researchers; and (3) at all times whilst engaging in the process, focus on the outcome – improving the quality of care for patients and their supporters.

References

Academy of Nursing, Midwifery and Health Visiting Research UK (undated) *The vision and mission of the Academy*. Available at: www.researchacademy.co.uk (accessed 1/7/2010).

Amsden, J and VanWynsberghe, R (2005) Community mapping as a research tool with youth. *Action Research* 3(4): 357–381. DOI: 10.1177/1476750305058487.

Baker, T A and Wang C (2006) Photovoice: Use of a participatory action research method to explore the chronic pain experience in older adults. *Qualitative Health Research* 16(10): 1405–1413. DOI: 10.1177/1049732306294118.

Beukema, L and Valkenburg, B (2007) Demand-driven elderly care in the Netherlands: A case exemplar in action research. *Action Research* 5(2): 161–180. DOI: 10.1177/1476750307077316.

Bridges, J and Meyer, J (2007) Exploring the effectiveness of action research as a tool for organizational change in health care. *Journal of Research in Nursing* 12: 389. DOI: 10.1177/1744987107078635.

Bridges, J, Meyer, J, Glynn, M, Bentley, J and Reeves, S (2003) Interprofessional care co-ordinators: The benefits and tensions associated with a new role in UK acute health care. *International Journal of Nursing Studies* 40(6): 599–607.

Brumley, D, Fisher, J, Robinson, H and Ashby, M (2006) Improving access to clinical information in after hours community palliative care. *Australian Journal of Advanced Nursing* 24(1): 27–31.

Buskens, I (2008) Research for change: Outcome mapping's contribution to emancipatory action research in Africa. *Action Research* 6(2): 171–192. DOI: 10.1177/1476750307087051.

Busza, J (2004) Participatory research in constrained settings:Sharing challenges from Cambodia. *Action Research* 2(2): 191–208. DOI: 10.1177/1476750304043730.

Chiu, LF (2003) Transformational potential of focus group practice in participatory action research. *Action Research* 1(2): 165–183. DOI: 10.1177/14767503030012006.

Choudhry, U K, Jandu, S, Mahal, J, Singh, R, Sohi-Pabla, H and Mutta, B (2004) Health promotion and participatory action research with South Asian women. *Journal of Nursing Scholarship* 34(1): 75–81. DOI 10.1111/j.1547-5069.2002.00075.x.

Cooper, J and Hewison, A (2002) Implementing audit in palliative care: An action research approach. *Journal of Advanced Nursing* 39(4): 360–369.

Day, J, Higgins, I and Koch T (2009) The process of practice redesign in delirium care for hospitalised older people: A participatory action research study. *International Journal of Nursing Studies* 46(1): 13–22.

de la Rue, M B (2003) Preventing ageism in nursing students: An action theory approach. *Australian Journal of Advanced Nursing* 20(4): 8–14.

Department of Health (2010) *Front-line care: The future of nursing and midwifery in England 2010*. The Prime Minister's Commission on the Future of Nursing and Midwifery in England. London: Department of Health/The Stationery Office. Available online at: http://cnm.independent.gov.uk (last accessed 24/11/2010).

Department of Health, Social Services and Public Safety (2010) *A partnership for care: Northern Ireland strategy for nursing and midwifery 2010–2015*. London: Department of Health/The Stationery Office. Available online at: www.dhsspsni.gov.uk/index/nmag/regional_nursing_and_midwifery_strategy-2.htm (accessed 24/11/2010).

Dickson, G (2008) Aboriginal grandmothers' experience with health promotion and participatory action research. *Action Research* 6(2): 171–192. DOI: 10.1177/1476750307087051.

Elsey, H and Lathlean, J (2006) Using action research to stimulate organisational change within health services: Experiences from two community-based studies. *Educational Action Research* 14(2): 171–186. DOI: 10.1080/09650790600718019.

Flicker, S, Maley, O, Ridgley, A, Biscope, S, Lombardo, C and Skinner HA (2008) e-PAR: Using technology and participatory action research to engage youth in health promotion. *Action Research* 6(3): 285–303. DOI: 10.1177/1476750307083711.

Fontana, J S (2004) A methodology for critical science in nursing. *Advances in Nursing Science* 27(2): 93–101.

Girot E A (2010) The challenges facing healthcare lecturers and professors to lead and promote a research-based culture for practice. *Journal of Research in Nursing* 15(3): 245–257.

Gray, D E (2009) *Doing research in the real world* (2nd edition). London: Sage.

Heslop, L, Elsom, S and Parker, N (2000) Improving continuity of care across psychiatric and emergency services: Combining patient data within a participatory action research framework. *Journal of Advanced Nursing* 31(1): 135–143.

Iversen, S, Ellertsen, B, Joacobsen, S R, Råheim, M and Knivsberg, A-M (2006) Developing a participatory multidisciplinary team approach to enhance the quality of school start. *Action Research* 4(3): 271–293. DOI: 10.1177/1476750306066802.

Jacobs, G (2006) Imagining the flowers, but working the rich and heavy clay: Participation and empowerment in action research for health. *Educational Action Research* 14(4): 569–581. DOI: 10.1080/09650790600975809.

Kelly, D and Simpson, S (2008) Action research in action: Reflections on a project to introduce clinical practice facilitators to an acute hospital setting. *Journal of Advanced Nursing* 33(5): 652–659. DOI: 10.1111/j.1365-2648.2001.01698.

Kemp, P (2000) Empowering the supporters: Enhancing the role of unqualified support workers in a housing scheme for people with mental health problems. *Educational Action Research*, 8(2): 261–275(15).

Kilgour, C and Fleming, V (2001) An action research inquiry into a health visitor parenting programme for parents of pre-school children with behaviour problems. *Journal of Advanced Nursing* 32(3): 682–688.

Khresheh, R and Barclay, L (2007) Practice–research engagement (PRE): Jordanian experience in three Ministry of Health hospitals. *Action Research* 5(2): 123–138. DOI: 10.1177/1476750307077313.

Koch, T and Kralik, D (2008) Chronic illness: Reflections on a community-based action research programme. *Journal of Advanced Nursing* 36(1): 23–31.

Lavie-Ajayi, M, Holmes, D and Jones, C (2007) 'We thought we "knew"', so we "did"': A voluntary organization's beginnings in action research. *Action Research* 5(4): 407–429. DOI: 10.1177/1476750307083719.

Lind, C (2007) The power of adolescent voices: Co-researchers in mental health promotion. *Educational Action Research* 15(3): 371–383. DOI: 10.1080/09650790701514309.

Liza, H and Elsom, S (2008) Improving continuity of care across psychiatric and emergency services: Combining patient data within a participatory action research framework. *Journal of Advanced Nursing* 31(1): 135–143.

Maiter, S, Simich, L, Jacobson, N and Wise, J (2008) Reciprocity: An ethic for community-based participatory action research. *Action Research* 6(3):305–325. DOI: 10.1177/1476750307083720.

McAllister, M and Stockhausen L (2001) Using action research within a school of nursing: Exposing tensions in ideologies. *Australian Journal of Advanced Nursing* 18(4): 15–22.

Mendenhall, T J and Doherty, W J (2007) Partners in diabetes: Action research in a primary care setting. *Action Research* 5(4): 378–406. DOI: 10.1177/1476750307083722.

Mills, J and Fitzgerald, M (2008) The changing role of practice nurses in Australia: An action research study. *Australian Journal of Advanced Nursing* 26(1): 16–20.

Nelson, G, Poland, B, Murray, M and Maticka-Tyndale, E (2004) Building capacity in community health action research: Towards a praxis framework for graduate education. *Action Research* 2(4): 389–408. DOI: 10.1177/1476750304047982.

Neuls, T (2003) Participating in action research on a health promotion project: A reflection. *Educational Action Research* 11(3): 415–428. DOI: 10.1080/09650790300200230.

NHS Education for Scotland (2009) *Nursing and midwifery education and workforce development: Towards 2020. Consensus Statement.* Available online at: www.nes.scot.nhs.uk/disciplines/nursing-and-midwifery (last accessed 11/10/2010).

Nomura, M, Makimoto, K, Kato, M, Shiba, T, Matsuura, C, Shigenobu, K, Ishikawa, T, Matsumoto, Nand Ikeda M (2009) Empowering older people with early dementia and family caregivers: A participatory action research study. *International Journal of Nursing Studies* 46(4): 431–441.

Philips, M E (2004) Action research and development coalitions in health care. *Action Research* 2(4): 349–370. DOI: 10.1177/1476750304047980.

Portillo, M C, Corchón, S, López-Dicastillo, O and Cowley S (2009) Evaluation of a nurse-led social rehabilitation programme for neurological patients and carers: An action research study. *International Journal of Nursing Studies* 46(2): 204–219.

Poulsen, K B, Jensen, S H, Bach, E and Schostak, J F (2007) Using action research to improve health and the work environment for 3,500 municipal bus drivers. *Educational Action Research* 15(1): 75–106.

Reid, R, Tom, A and Frisby W (2006) Finding the 'action' in feminist participatory action research. *Action Research* 4(3): 315–332. DOI: 10.1177/1476750306066804.

Rycroft-Malone J and Burton C (2010) Paying attention to complexity in implementation research. Editorial. *Worldviews on Evidence-Based Nursing* 7(3) : 121–122. DOI: 10.1111/j.1741-6787.2010.00200.x.

Stead, V, Mort, M and Davies, J (2001) Theory generation and practice improvement: A mental health service perspective. *Educational Action Research* 9(1): 61–77. DOI: 10.1080/09650790100200145.

Stuttaford, M and Coe, C (2007) The 'learning' component of participatory learning and action in health research: Reflections from a local Sure Start evaluation. *Qualitative Health Research* 17(10): 1351–1360. DOI: 10.1177/1049732307306965.

Teram, E, Schachter, CL and Stalker, CA (2005) The case for integrating grounded theory and participatory action research: Empowering clients to inform professional practice. *Qualitative Health Research* 15(8): 1129–1140. DOI: 10.1177/1049732305275882.

Vallenga, D, Grypdonck, M H F, Tan, F I Y, Lendemeijer, B H G M and Boon, P A J M (2008) Improving decision-making in caring for people with epilepsy and intellectual disability: An action research project. *Journal of Advanced Nursing* 61(3): 261–272.

Vatne, S, Bjornerem, H and Hoem, E (2009) Development of professional knowledge in action: Experiences from an action science design focusing on acknowledging communication in mental health. *Scandinavian Journal of Caring Sciences* 23(1): 84–92. DOI: 10.1111/j.1471-6712.2007.00593.x

Wai-tong Chien, W, Wai-chi Chan, S and Morrissey, J (2002) The use of learning contracts in mental health nursing clinical placement: An action research. *International Journal of Nursing Studies* 39(7): 685–694.

Waterman, H, Harker, R, MacDonald, H, McLaughlan, R and Waterman, C (2005a) Evaluation of an action research project in ophthalmic nursing practice. *Journal of Advanced Nursing* 52(4): 389–398. DOI 10.1111/j.1365-2648.2005.03606.x.

Waterman, H, Harker, R, MacDonald, H, McLaughlan, R and Waterman, C (2005b) Advancing ophthalmic nursing practice through action research. *Journal of Advanced Nursing* 52(3): 281–290. DOI 10.1111/j.1365-2648.2005.03594.

Waterman, H, Marshall, M, Noble, J, Davies, H, Walshe, K, Sheaff, R and Elwyn, G (2007) The role of action research in the investigation and diffusion of innovations in health care: The PRIDE project. *Qualitative Health Research* 17(3): 373–381. DOI: 10.1177/1049732306298976.

Welsh Assembly Government (2009) *The Post-registration framework*. Cardiff: Welsh Assembly. Available online at: http://wales.gov.uk/docs/phhs/consultation/career framework/090924reporten.pdf (last accessed 24/11/2010).

Westhues, A, Ochocka J, Jacobson, N, Simich, L, Maiter, S, Janzen, R and Fleras, A (2008) Developing theory from complexity: Reflections on a collaborative mixed method participatory action research study. *Qualitative Health Research* 18(5): 701–717. DOI: 10.1177/1049732308316531.

Whitehead, D (2005) Commentary on Walsgrove H and Fulbrook P (2005) Advancing the clinical perspective: A practice development project to develop the nurse practitioner role in an acute hospital trust. *Journal of Clinical Nursing* 12, 444–455. *Journal of Clinical Nursing* 148): 1032.

Williamson, G R and Prosser, S (2002) Action research: Politics, ethics and participation. *Journal of Advanced Nursing* 40(5): 587–593.

Williamson, G R, Webb, C and Abelson-Mitchell, N (2004) Developing lecturer practitioner roles using action research. *Journal of Advanced Nursing* 47(2): 153–164.

GLOSSARY

Backfill Contract staff are brought in to replace permanent staff who are engaged in long-term work, for example, in Chapter 4, as clinical action research facilitator co-researcher.

Democratic Originating in ancient Greek politics, a democratic form of government is one in which citizens elect other citizens to represent their views and make laws following discussion and debate. In action research it is used to indicate that consensus and ongoing discussion are in evidence.

Dialectic This is a term with a long history in philosophy and with roots in ancient Greek thought, in which opposing viewpoints are presented and discussed, leading to changes in the understanding of the arguments and directions in which they develop. Understanding is thus made up of different viewpoints, and change occurs when one viewpoint gains an upper hand (as a result of dialogue) and influences the way in which thought develops. In philosophy, dialectic processes take place when thesis (a viewpoint) meets antithesis (its opposing viewpoint) , and the resulting exchange leads to synthesis (a new way of understanding).

Emancipation A political definition is to set free or liberate oneself or others from some condition or situation which is unjust or oppressive in some way. There is an imbalance of power between those who control the situation and those seeking liberation that needs to be overcome for emancipation to occur.

Experiment in research, an experiment is a term used (in contemporary healthcare) where a new intervention (such as a new medication) is introduced to participants (patients) to measure effectiveness against a placebo or existing treatments. Randomised controlled trials are one example of these in healthcare research. The term is not generally used within contemporary clinical action research because of the nature and importance of collaboration, stakeholder involvement coupled with participation, joint working and learning.

Feminism A political movement seeking women's emancipation from the oppression of men and society.

Hermeneutic In research, this is a paradigm distinct from a positivist approach. Hermeneutics seeks to interpret and understand human experience and holds that such experience is not fixed but is always changing.

Hypertension High blood pressure.

Hypothesis A hypothesis theory or premise. Used in positivist research as a means of showing ideas that are to be proved or disproved in the research study.

Interpretivism A school of thought associated with critical theory and anti-positivism which rejects the idea that human experience can be understood by collecting empirical scientific data and instead that human culture, norms and values are important.

Knowledge-constitutive paradigms A term associated with the critical theorist Jürgen Habermas meaning ways by which knowledge and understanding of social life are constructed in the social as well as the physical sciences.

Lifeworld processes A term originating with Habermas which means the processes by which we communicate and are socialised. His theory of communicative action holds that free dialogue between individuals is more important to emancipation than economic power, and in contemporary societies oppression now comes from centralised mass media.

Natural sciences These are the physical sciences, such as physics, biology and chemistry, as distinct from the social sciences such as sociology and psychology.

Outcome evaluation Identifying the extent to which the project's objectives have been achieved, the learning that has taken place, and the identification of ways to sustain the project.

Paradigm A model or a worldview of something. In research there is the qualitative paradigm, quantitative paradigm and critical paradigm.

Political acumen The sharpness of mind and the ability to make quick, accurate, intelligent judgements about people or situations in organisations.

Positivism A school of thought developed in the nineteenth century by Auguste Comte and others which sees scientific methods of inquiry as the only way of establishing the underlying processes in human society. Testable hypotheses rather than philosophical speculation are essential for understanding the facts of social life; it is a viewpoint heavily influenced by the natural sciences. A founding principle of quantitative research.

Process evaluation This determines the extent to which the project is moving forward; it identifies the drivers and barriers to change and the issues still to be addressed.

Reflexivity In social research, this means a researcher's acknowledgement that they have had an impact on the research setting, and the setting has also had an impact on the researcher. This is particularly important in action research where the researcher is also a participant. It enables the action researcher to lay bare and make explicit their thinking in relation to the research study and setting.

Validity In research, **validity** can mean that an instrument or item measures what it is supposed to measure. In action research, it means whether the research is truthful and appropriate.

INDEX